AUTOPHAGY

HOW TO COMBINE INTERMITTENT FASTING AND
NOBEL-PRIZE WINNING SCIENCE FOR RAPID
WEIGHT LOSS, REDUCING INFLAMMATION, AND
PROMOTING LONG-TERM HEALTH

THOMAS HAWTHORN

Thomas Hawthorn

© Copyright 2019 - All rights reserved.

The following Book is reproduced below with the goal of providing information that is as accurate and reliable as possible. Regardless, purchasing this eBook can be seen as consent to the fact that both the publisher and the author of this book are in no way experts on the topics discussed within and that any recommendations or suggestions that are made herein are for entertainment purposes only. Professionals should be consulted as needed prior to undertaking any of the action endorsed herein.

This declaration is deemed fair and valid by both the American Bar Association and the Committee of Publishers Association and is legally binding throughout the United States.

Furthermore, the transmission, duplication or reproduction of any of the following work including specific information will be considered an illegal act irrespective of if it is done electronically or in print. This extends to creating a secondary or tertiary copy of the work or a recorded copy and is only allowed with an expressed written consent from the Publisher. All additional right reserved.

The information in the following pages is broadly considered to be a truthful and accurate account of facts and as such any inattention, use or misuse of the information in question by the reader will render any resulting actions solely under their purview. There are no scenarios in which the publisher or the original author of this work can be in any fashion deemed liable for any hardship or damages that may befall them after undertaking information described herein.

Additionally, the information in the following pages is intended only for informational purposes and should thus be thought of as universal. As befitting its nature, it is presented without assurance regarding its prolonged validity or interim quality. Trademarks that are mentioned are done without written consent and can in no way be considered an endorsement from the trademark holder.

Medical Disclaimer

This book is not intended as a substitute for the medical advice of physicians. The reader should regularly consult a physician in matters relating to his/her health and particularly with respect to any symptoms that may require diagnosis or medical attention.

Please consult your physician before starting any diet or exercise program.

Any recommendations given in this book are not a substitute for medical advice.

❧ Created with Vellum

INTRODUCTION

*I*t is time to cell-destruct!

BUT BEFORE I explain that statement, perhaps I should give you a little bit of background. So, let's start with that.

AUTOPHAGY IS the newest lifestyle habit to take the world by storm. As more people become aware of the benefits of autophagy, more people adopt the process as a permanent part of their lives.

THEY START FOLLOWING the techniques of autophagy ardently. They change their diet, alter their habits, and curb down on all those morning frappuccinos and extra-sugary foods.

THEY START LIVING HEALTHILY.

. . .

When individuals adopt the healthy lifestyle of autophagy, you can notice visible changes in them. They become more active and have a certain 'glow' (which is actually the body gaining back its vitality). They are even more productive and focused on their tasks.

I know you are probably thinking about the diet fads that you may have seen on TV or while browsing online. Your first impression is probably one of mistrust.

Let me tell you, though, that everything you are about to read here is backed up by science and heavy research. There have been actual scientific reports that have been conducted to support the process of autophagy and how it can benefit us.

However, no one likes to read a lengthy medical exposition.

If there is one thing that can put people off about a subject is the use of complex terms that don't make any sense. Or even if they do make sense, it is only because someone has taken the time to Google the terminology while reading. In fact, most books contain enough medical terms to give anybody their Ph.D. in Medicine. So, we will try and avoid this and keep things as simple as possible.

Even if I have to support some arguments with science, I will make it easy for you to grasp the complexities of every topic in the book.

This is not going to be a medical journal that you will not be able to understand.

. . .

You will realize how autophagy can benefit your life and give you one of the keys to a healthy lifestyle.

In this book, you will see how autophagy destroys harmful cells and brings back some of the vigor in your life.

Science will be used to back up the statements, that are going to be presented in a way that's easy to understand.

You are about to venture on a healthy journey that is not merely based on theories and suppositions and should change your life for the better.

Your ideas about dieting will also change as we show you the ways in which autophagy takes care of excess fats waiting to be used for energy.

So, let us get started on this journey of self-healing and better living.

It is time for you to receive the gift of autophagy that your body has been trying to bless you with for your whole life.

AUTOPHAGY IN PLAIN ENGLISH

When our ancestors were hunting and gathering, they were not aware of when they would get to eat next. Their bodies saw this situation as a threat and tried to protect themselves when there was no food to provide the necessary nutrients. In such situations, their systems dealt with stress and went through a cleansing process after hours of not receiving any sustenance.

WHEN THE CLEANSING OCCURRED, the body would target damaged and dangerous cells, which could harm the body by turning cancerous. What this meant was that our ancestors' bodies developed to fit a state of fasting. During that period, their system would aim to help instead of harming itself.

ACCORDING to the US National Library of Medicine National Institutes of Health, it is not natural for people to have three meals a day.

. . .

IT IS NOT a part of our evolutionary design at all. More surprisingly, it does not provide any additional benefits to the body.

ALTHOUGH PEOPLE TEND to feel hungry if and when they skip lunch, that hunger occurs due to certain habits. For a long time, after all, we have trained ourselves to receive food in the afternoons. When our body gets hungry, though, it does not entail that it has no nutrition or energy. That is merely its way of reacting to a habit that we have established previously.

CAUSES OF AUTOPHAGY

IF YOU LOOK through the vast library of the US National Library of Medicine National Institutes of Health, then you might find the solution to that. In a nutshell, it has got to do with a particular protein named p62.

THE P62 PROTEIN identifies harmful cell waste, which is then cleared off by a process known as autophagy. It basically tells the body to "eat" the harmful cells. Without the identification process for this protein, your system will never recognize the harm caused by its own cells.

IN ESSENCE, the presence of p62 is one of the many factors responsible for a healthy and improved lifestyle of people. So, yes, autophagy is extremely good for the body. However, there are more benefits to the process than the mere removal of bad cells.

AUTOPHAGY HELPS in regulating the levels of inflammation.

Here is something you should know about inflammation: it is not always easy to detect, especially when it becomes chronic.

CHRONIC INFLAMMATION TAKES place in the form of various side effects, such as rashes, pain, swelling, red skin and other symptoms. Sometimes, it can stay dormant in your body and may not present any symptoms until decades later. It may just surprise you when you least expect it.

AUTOPHAGY MAKES several contributions to our immune system. Because it has numerous roles to play, they are combined together under one field of study, which is known as immunophagy.

WHEN AUTOPHAGY BECOMES ACTIVE, it performs a plethora of tasks that reduce inflammation. Let us look at a few of them:

- Autophagy reduces the build-up of proteins that cause inflammation. In other words, it prevents the process from getting worse.
- Crohn's disease is a common illness that causes inflammation of the bowel system. Basically, it is a type of IBD that you have learned about in the previous chapter. When you activate autophagy, the process prevents the disease from spreading. In fact, autophagy is an essential component of the treatment of Crohn's, and hence, you should focus on a diet that activates autophagy.
- One of the proteins that cause inflammation is called nuclear factor kappa-light-chain-enhancer of activated B cells (NFKB). The name is mouthful indeed, but let's say that the excess of this protein simply spells bad news. Where does autophagy come into this? Well, the process

reduces the levels of NFKB in the body. This, in turn, reduces inflammation levels.

When autophagy takes over, it not only curbs the harmful effects of inflammation but also provides these benefits to the body:

- You may notice that your bodily functions begin to improve. You feel less lethargic and more active as well.
- Damaged cells harm your body to such an extent that it impacts longevity. After all, you are living with cells that have already degraded or are degrading at a faster rate. This means that parts of the body do not function with the same vitality as they have had before. With autophagy, though, you are replacing the old, harmful, and useless cells with healthier ones. This helps your body to work with renewed vitality, as well as allow you to act and feel younger. When that happens, you are practically enhancing your longevity.
- We have already seen a number of diseases that take place due to inflammation. Autophagy can help manage or prevent them and even delay numerous neurodegenerative conditions.

"Neurodegenerative diseases" is basically an umbrella term that describes a host of conditions that affect the neurons in the brain. If you have heard of illnesses like Alzheimer's, Parkinson's, or Huntington's, then you should realize that they all fall under this category.

THESE DISEASES HAVE a profound effect on the individual and their daily functions. For example, Alzheimer's causes the gradual degradation of a person's memory. In many cases, the people suffering from these diseases experience confusion with respect to time and space.

. . .

Regardless of the neurodegenerative disease that you are at risk of facing, though, autophagy can help you avoid falling prey to the illness or slow down its advancement at least.

Activating Autophagy

We have understood that autophagy is good. Now, how can we activate it? Also, what can we do to help our body rid itself of the bad cells, feel rejuvenated, and help you lead a healthy and long life?

Before we delve into that, you should know a few things first. The most important one is the fact that a study on autophagy has received the Nobel Prize. In 2016, to be specific, a Japanese cell biologist named Yoshinori Ohsumi was given the award for his work on how the body recycles content.[1] Apparently, it breaks down proteins and other components that it considers nonessential and then uses them for energy. This process was named - you guessed it - autophagy. It comes from a blend of two words in Greek: "auto" (meaning self) and "phagy" (meaning to eat).

The definition of the word is not far from the truth. In fact, the body is practically consuming the bad cells to prevent them from causing harm. In the process, it gains energy, which is used for its daily functions.

Still, the recycling procedure goes further than simply getting rid of nonessential substances. Ohsumi has discovered that some cells use the process of autophagy to get rid of viruses and bacteria by sending them to get recycled. This way, the body not only gains energy afterward but also ends up removing the harmful foreign bodies. Further research has shown that interferences in autophagy have an effect on its aging process. This means that if you want to live healthier (and longer), you need to let the body eat all the harmful cells that are accumulating within it.

All of these discoveries on autophagy have raised a very important question: When does the process become active?

Thankfully, science has an answer to that.

Self-Eating

When the body does not receive food, it begins to eat itself. It does not do this in such a horrifying way that you might just think of it as a concept for a horror movie. No, this is not the X-Files we are talking about. This is a natural process that the body has honed over millenniums. It started with our ancestors who lived in caves.

When you fast, restrict calories, and go on a diet, you are encouraging our body to activate autophagy.

You are encouraging your body to start its regenerative transformation.

Of course, one of the questions that many people ask is: Doesn't the body get rid of nonessential cells anyways? Why do we need autophagy?

. . .

The reason is that, as we age, we experience stress, change in diet, physical stagnation, and other pressures that life throws at us. This speeds up the rate at which our cells begin to break down. Add to that our habit of feeding our body unhealthy components; then we have essentially created a recipe for disaster.

This is where autophagy comes in. Using the process, the body focuses on removing the ever-increasing number of deteriorating cells, including the senescent cells that provide no use to the body other than moving around inside organs and tissues. Nevertheless, even though senescent cells do not have any use, they are still capable of causing harm. These can activate inflammatory pathways and could become vital factors in the formation of various diseases. We just don't need them and, thankfully, we have autophagy to get rid of them.

Is there a way to activate the autophagy process by yourself? Sure, there is. There are five different ways to make sure that you can achieve that. However, you should know that you cannot depend on one method alone. You have to ensure that each of them is used with the remaining techniques in the list.

Method 1: Low-Carb Diet

The first thing that you should focus on is taking care of those extra carbs that go into your body. Carbohydrates have low-fiber content and can be digested easily. When you eat them, they cause a major imbalance in the sugar levels of the body. To be specific, the blood sugar levels drop quickly after having a meal that is rich in carbs. In fact, you can start noticing changes within an hour or two, making you feel hungry more quickly.

. . .

You end up feeling like you have not eaten anything filling. To make sure you keep your hunger at bay, you need to consume more food, eventually increasing the carb intake and putting on extra pounds. Before you know it, your weight has gone up drastically, and you are unsure how it has happened!

Furthermore, all the sugar that you have consumed gets stored as fat, even though they are not doing anything. They are simply there. It is like hoarding your house with boxes of canned food and letting them just sit there and do nothing. However, having too many canned foods at home does not cause it to expand or bloat. Your body, on the other hand, functions a little more differently, considering the more fats that accumulate inside, the more it begins to expand.

And we all know where this is going: increased weight and body mass. That' not a good combination.

When you decrease your carb intake, then you are essentially forcing your body to go into hunger mode. Just remember (as you have read about before) that this sensation is produced not because you do not get enough nutrients. A more likely reason is that your body is used to having food at certain times. So, when you do not eat, it simply asks you to consume more food.

Nevertheless, this time, you are going to refuse it, especially if you want to induce autophagy and burn those extra fats.

Method 2: High-Fat Diet

Now, don't get me wrong. I am not saying that fats are bad. Rather, it is the kind of fats that you consume that you should be worried about.

You see, you can get healthy fats from various sources. They help the body receive more energy, which is vital for activating autophagy that involves going into fasting mode. You will remove all the sources of carbs and sugar into your life, and that causes hunger pangs to crop up regularly. You are going to prevent the body from trying to seek out energy from sources of carbs, so you need to take energy from other sources.

What you should do is concentrate on obtaining fats from fruits, vegetables, nuts, eggs, and other healthier alternatives. However, you cannot keep on taking these fats. You need to schedule a particular point in the day in which you are going to break your fast with a healthy, high-fat meal.

Once you have consumed that food, you should head back into a fast to begin to burn away all those carbs. By keeping this method of fasting as a routine, you are forcing your body to flush out the carbohydrates stored in it. You are teaching it to depend on the fats alone as its source of energy.

Method 3: Intermittent Fasting

People often pose a question about fasting: Isn't it similar to starvation?

. . .

THE ANSWER: not even close.

WHEN YOU ARE FASTING, you are doing something that does not occur during starvation: you are exerting control. When you starve, after all, food is involuntarily unavailable to you for a long time. This causes a lot of suffering too. Besides, nothing about starvation is deliberate. You are not doing it because it is beneficial for you.

WHEN YOU FAST, you are choosing to withhold the food that is supplied to your body in a controlled manner. Yes, it is true that you do feel hungry, but that is because of body habits (as we have seen earlier). You fast because you participate in a health or spiritual process.

IN THE CASE of fasting as well, you have food readily available. You can eat anytime you want. However, you choose not to do so. Additionally, there is no fixed time for fasting. You can fast for a few hours up to an entire day. The whole point of the method is to make sure that you bring about positive changes in your body.

THAT IS WHY THE TERM 'BREAKFAST' exists. You are essentially breaking a fast. In a normal situation, you typically have dinner in the evening, followed by an 8- or 9-hour sleep before having breakfast. That particular gap is your fasting period. During such a time, your body takes care of vital processes in your body. When you finally decide to eat food, the body takes all the important nutrients from the meal.

THIS IS the main purpose of intermittent fasting as well. You are not depriving yourself of food. Instead, you are teaching your body to rely on meals when you provide it.

. . .

Let us examine everything that we have understood by looking at what happens while fasting.

When we eat, the levels of insulin in our body increases. Then, the body breaks down the carbohydrates into single sugar units, which combine together to form long chains that are called glycogen. The glycogen is stored in the muscle or liver; that's why you have a source of energy to tap into when you need it!

Now, what's the catch, you ask?

Here is what happens. The storage space for carbohydrates is not unlimited. When it reaches the limit, then any excess is then converted to fat. A part of this newly created fat is stored in the liver. However, a large portion of it gets diverted to other areas of the body, most particularly in the fat deposits. Hence, you begin to notice the expansion of numerous parts of the body as fats accumulate in them.

When we start fasting, the insulin levels fall. This is a signal for the body to begin burning all the stored fat. In fact, at this point, the glucose levels in the blood also start to drop. The body is then forced to consume the extra fat it has stored before.

The result is that you begin to lose weight.

When you look at the way the body works when it comes to storing fat, you may notice two distinct scenarios. One is that when you eat constantly, you supply food in your body at every opportunity. This increases the fat reserves without burning the ones that are already there.

THE OTHER THING is that you should not indulge the body throughout the day. You should only eat at a particular time and make sure to avoid the three-meals-a-day plan. This forces the body to use up all the stored fats and depend on them to obtain energy.

THINK ABOUT IT; which situation would you like to adopt into your life?

METHOD 4: Exercise

WHEN OUR ANCESTORS used to hunt animals and discovered new sources of food, they were always on the move. They would keep their bodies active as much as possible.

THIS TECHNIQUE ALLOWED them to stay fit, and a balance was created. The food provided our ancestors with energy. The hunting and gathering activities, on the other hand, helped them to dispense that energy. Unbeknownst to them, they had found the ideal way to live healthily.

FAST FORWARD TO THE PRESENT, we are not hunting in the forests for food while wearing deerskins anymore. Instead, we are busy hunting the shelves of the local stores for all the food with high amount of carbohydrates. Our only source of activity lies in the small tasks that we engage in every day as well. Still, they are not enough to expend the energy stored in our bodies. We need to be more active. Thus, exercises have become a thing.

WHAT WE ARE DOING IS USING physical activities to burn away calories. When you combine exercise with fasting and a proper diet, you not only provide your body with good nutrients and fats but also ensure that no fat gets deposited in places where they do not belong. You are only storing enough fats for your body to utilize; you are not keeping excess fats, which lead to more harmful side effects, health-wise.

EXERCISE CAN BE DONE in many ways. You can swim, jog, walk briskly, dance, or skip. Alternatively, you can head over to the gym and go through some high-intensity workout routines. The choice is entirely up to you. The key thing to remember is that when you are exercising, you should not do it occasionally. You have to make it a habit. Nevertheless, there is more to exercise than just burning fats.

WHEN YOU WORKOUT, after all, it results in changes in the brain that lower levels of stress and depression. In a study mentioned in the US National Library of Medicine National Institutes of Health, 24 women who were diagnosed with depression began displaying fewer signs of depression after doing regular exercises. In another study, 26 men and women who were exercising regularly were brought in for an experiment. Some of them were asked to stop exercising while others were allowed to continue their routines. It turned out that those who stopped working out noticed an increase in their negative moods.

ON THE OTHER HAND, exercises also helped develop the muscles and bones, so you were getting both a physical and mental workout. But the real question lies in how. To be specific, how does exercise help the muscles and the bones in our body? When you exercise, you release hormones that improve the ability of your muscles to absorb amino acids, which are responsible for reducing the breakdown of muscles and improving their growth. When it comes to bones, exercise helps to boost their density.

WORKING out also increases everyone's energy level. With better metabolism, your body is able to use energy better and distribute it to various parts of the body. It is like transferring electricity to different areas in your house; you are making sure that no room has to remain in the dark. You can use a similar concept when it comes to exercising to feel active and ready to perform physical tasks.

Now, I would like you to take a look at the benefits mentioned above. What would be the best process to complement your exercise routines? What could help get the most perks out of your physical activities?

YOU KNOW THE ANSWER. Autophagy, of course.

AUTOPHAGY AND EXERCISE

WHEN YOU COMBINE autophagy with exercise, you are taking a powerful combination to bring your body back to good health. Developing your muscles and bones? Let autophagy take care of the waste. Trying to get more energy? Autophagy can remove the harmful fat cells that accumulate in the body and help you store healthy fat for energy.

. . .

No matter what benefit you may want to derive from your exercises, autophagy can make things much better.

But what else can autophagy achieve? How does it create all the advantages it comes with? It is time to delve deeper into that and answer some of those pertinent "how" questions.

Let's look at the short- and long-term benefits of autophagy.

HIGHLY INFLAMMABLE: WHY INFLAMMATION IS KILLING YOU

*A*ccording to the National Human Genome Research Institute, nearly 99% of the genetic makeup of all human beings are the same.

IT LEAVES JUST 1% for differences in human beings to create all the variation that we see amongst our species.

THIS SMALL PERCENTAGE of variation allows unique physiological diversities, which lead to different skin tones, eye colors, hair colors, body masses, and other features to develop in humans.

We notice these changes in the people around us; all you have to do is take a step outside to see that. Even if you are living within a small community, the unique features between each individual will still be evident.

THE THING IS, that the 1% difference between us is what scientists are interested in.

. . .

To researchers and scientists, the small percentage of uniqueness each human being has, helps them discover the cause of various diseases and other problems that can affect people.

Their discoveries help them focus on identifying and forming solutions to illnesses and various medical problems. They then create new prescription drugs, procedures, and other preventive measures.

While drugs and different treatments are all beneficial to us, scientists have discovered something more interesting.

Simply changing your diet, you can prevent and hold off a myriad of medical problems and keep numerous diseases at bay.

Scientists have brought to light the idea that modifying dietary and fitness plans can delay the onset of type 2 diabetes, even in people who carry a predisposition for this condition.

This opens up new doors into dietary research and, provides an answer to the misconception that dieting only works for some people.

There has been an increase in various dieting plans and techniques around the world in the last 20 years, so it's no wonder people are confused about what to do.

. . .

NEVERTHELESS, dieting is important? And this book will endeavour to make the dieting process easier and simpler than ever before.

NO MATTER what diet you chose in the future, autophagy will be part of the formula that makes losing weight and being healthier easier than you ever imagined.

UNDERSTANDING *Inflammation*

Simply put, it is your body's response to external factors such as infections, stress, foreign bodies, or even toxins that pose a threat to you.

When your immune system detects any of them, it releases certain proteins that are made to protect tissues and cells.

IT DOES NOT SOUND SO bad does it? It actually sounds like the body is doing something good and it is.

IN THE CASE of the above example, inflammation is indeed useful as your body uses its defence mechanisms to fight infections, diseases, and other foreign bodies.

HOWEVER, in numerous cases, the process can work against us. This means that when we consume fatty and sugary foods, the process of inflammation may not be beneficial to us.

WHEN YOU ARE CONSUMING a high amount of fat (and not the good fats, which we shall see later) and sugar, you are forcing your system to activate the inflammation.

. . .

At this point, your immune cells tend to react for no apparent reason other than the intake of substances like fats and sugar.

This is when the problems begin to occur.

∼

Gut Punch!
Many of your immune cells congregate in your intestines. When your body feels like it has to release your immune cells, it does so in appropriate doses, enough to fight the threat that seeks to harm the body. During this time, they ignore the healthy bacteria that reside in your gut.

When you force your body into the inflammation process, then your immune system attacks your gut, especially the digestive tract. This creates an autoimmune response called inflammatory bowel disease (IBD). This refers to a situation in which your body's immune responses become your own enemy. Meaning, the antibodies begin to attack healthy tissues and cells.

Imagine losing control over your own body's defence functions. It's not a good feeling.

Joint Venture

When inflammations occur, they target different parts of the body. If your diet causes inflammation in the joints, though, it can lead to some serious damage. One of the conditions that you can suffer from is known as rheumatoid arthritis (RA).

. . .

ACCORDING to a study conducted at the Yale School of Medicine, a salt-heavy diet can cause multiple autoimmune diseases such as psoriasis (a chronic skin condition), multiple sclerosis (reduction of the protective covering around your nerves), and of course, rheumatoid arthritis (chronic inflammation of the joints).

NOT HALE and Hearty

ANY PART of your body can kickstart the inflammation process, even your heart. When fat begins to clog arteries, they can attract your white blood cells. The white blood cells then crowd your arteries further. Then, your heart is just a few cells away from a heart attack.

RISK OF CANCER

THAT'S RIGHT.
Based on a study conducted at the Harvard Medical School, inflammatory diets (that include fats and sugar) promote colorectal cancer. Worse, if the inflammation becomes chronic, the risk of developing cervical, lung, and oesophageal cancers may increase. With that said, eating a lot of hotdogs, sugars, and junk foods is not the best choice for your body.

IT MAY BE Bad for Your Lungs

INFLAMMATION CAN OCCUR ANYWHERE in the body. This means that your lungs are not safe from its effects as well. In reality, the results of inflammation in the lungs are rather severe. It can cause the accumulation of fluid in the airways, for instance, which limit the supply of air to your lungs. Eventually, you might find yourself having difficulty in breathing.

ADDITIONALLY, diseases such as asthma are linked to the inflammation of the lungs.

Gum Control

WHEN YOUR GUMS ARE INFLAMED, the bacteria begin to accumulate around your teeth. This causes periodontitis, a disease in which your gums begin to recede. Furthermore, the strong skeletal structure that supports them grow weak and may suffer damage easily. You will eventually have to endure teeth sensitivity, among other problems.

TIME FOR A **CRP**

IF YOU THOUGHT that I meant to say CPR and just made a spelling error, then you should know that that's not the case at all. I am not asking you to go through an emergency procedure to bring back your breathing. Instead, I am talking about the c-reactive protein (CRP) test.

ESSENTIALLY, what this test does is to check the levels of c-reactive proteins in your body. These proteins are released into your bloodstream when inflammation takes place. The more c-reactive proteins you have, the higher the degree of inflammation will be. If your CRP levels are more than 350 milligrams per litre, then you have to consider the fact that you may have a condition that requires immediate medical care.

If you want to discover the CRP levels in your body, you should get in touch with your doctor to understand the inflammation levels of your body. If they happen to be higher than usual, then your physician may give you medications or therapies to lower the levels of CRP in your body.

However, rather than focusing on heading to the doctor, it might perhaps be the right time to change your diet.

A key thing to remember is that even if you have normal levels of inflammation in your body, it does not mean that it cannot increase in the future. Which is why, you need to make sure that you focus on a healthier way of eating and living.

The Solution

Your body follows a natural process when it comes to dealing with threats. It understands how to react to danger and targets the problem with efficiency. When your body turns against you, though, the results are not only catastrophic but also demoralizing. Imagine realizing that your body is not protecting you anymore and is focused on harming you instead.

Nonetheless, all it takes is a good diet to bring about positive changes within yourself. The benefits that come with it are not mere speculations. They are facts established by the scientific community.

THOMAS HAWTHORN

. . .

AT THIS POINT, you may be wondering if there is a diet that can align your body on the path of good health. Is there one that can prevent your system from causing inflammation when it is not supposed to?

AS IT TURNS OUT, there is, and we are just about to get to know more about it. But first, let's talk a little about autophagy.

THE LONG AND SHORT OF IT: FINDING THE LONG-TERM AND SHORT-TERM BENEFITS OF AUTOPHAGY

We have briefly touched upon the benefits of autophagy. While they definitely showed the significance of autophagy to the body, they were not explored in detailed. You see, there are more ways for you to take advantage of this process. Take metabolism for example.

When you think about it, autophagy is like taking out the trash in our body. When it does that, it ends up replacing parts of the cells, including the mitochondria. Simply put, these are the engines - the powerhouse - of your cells. They help your body to burn fat and make adenosine triphosphate (ATP), a complex substance that provides energy for various processes that take place in the cells.

There are a lot of harmful toxic materials in the mitochondria that can cause harm to the cells. Is it important to remove or break down their build up so that they cannot cause the fast aging of the cells. When autophagy takes over, it helps use the toxic substances as energy instead. This helps to prevent them from spreading as well. Eventually, the body receives more fuel and has the resources to make more proteins that can bring back the life into our cells.

THE TRUTH IS that we all need healthy cells. They are essential for improving your metabolism. Thus, your body can function better. Of course, convincing people about autophagy is a challenge in itself. When people are told about it, they often respond with disbelief.

THAT IS an understandable reaction if I have to be honest. Imagine telling someone that you know a process that can actually reduce the occurrence of Alzheimer's disease. People might look at you as though you just sprouted a second head. However, you may be able to convince them by explaining just how it makes these wonderful changes in the body.

So, let us try to see if we can work out some of the details behind the many claims of autophagy.

Reducing the Risk of Neurodegenerative Diseases: How?

MANY OF THE neurodegenerative diseases (including the ones that have been mentioned earlier) develop because of complex proteins in the brain cells stop functioning correctly. As always, the reason behind their malfunction can be anything from aging to poor diet. Some of these diseases take time to manifest because the proteins that stop working properly begin to accumulate, and they do so rather slowly. When more of them gathers, the illness that's waiting to get activated finds all the capability to do so. Eventually, you are left with a brain that becomes tormented by a host of symptoms.

. . .

Because autophagy helps clean damaged cells, though, it can help the brain rid itself of the proteins that act like a ticking time bomb. For example, the process can eliminate amyloid, a protein that is deposited in various parts of the body when you have Alzheimer's. It removes the alpha-synuclein as well, which is activated by Parkinson's disease.

By merely focusing on a specific protein, autophagy makes sure that any neurodegenerative disease does affect your brain or cause as much harm as it normally does.

Prevent Cancer Onset: *How?*

Autophagy can subdue certain processes that can lead to cancer, such as DNA damage response and genome instability. What this means is that any damaged protein that cause instability in our genes or prevent our body from repairing damaged DNA gets flushed out of the system. While conducting research on mice, scientists discovered that the rodents with poor autophagy showed increased rates of cancer.

Improves Skin Health: *How?*

The skin is the largest organ in the body and is one that is exposed to the elements a lot. When the cells underneath are exposed to these elements, then they take face the harmful effects from air pollution, chemicals, humidity changes, cold and hot weather, and even physical impacts. All of that beating is bound to have some effect on the cells!

...

In truth, the cells begin to age quickly due to that, so your skin looks older than it should. Autophagy works on these cells. Any cell that does not function well is recycled, but if there are cells that can still be used, then the process makes them work efficiently. This contributes to healthier looking skin.

When people comment about how someone's skin glows, they are probably talking about how autophagy has contributed to an improved cell function.

If you look at skin cells, they always have a tough time preventing bacteria from entering the body. When they work, it is important to support them so that they are not doing all the heavy lifting alone.

Guess what they need? Yup, a heavy dose of help from our good friend autophagy.

Prevents Extreme Cell Death: How?

Your body actually makes cells die. It is a programmed function that occurs to everyone. It is not caused by a particular disease or genetic disorder.

In other words, your cells commit suicide in a process known as apoptosis.

...

AUTOPHAGY

WHEN YOU ANALYZE autophagy and apoptosis, then you are looking at processes with similar goals: to remove damaged cells from the body. What separates the two aside from the way they work - autophagy recycles cells while apoptosis makes cells destroy themselves - is their results.

WHEN AUTOPHAGY TAKES PLACE, the cells are recycled and used for energy or flushed out of the system. On the other hand, when apoptosis takes over, then you are looking at a lot of wasted cells in the body. It is much like cleaning out the house but leaving the trash inside. Yeah, definitely disgusting.

IN ORDER TO clean up the mess, the body uses another process: inflammation. We have just seen how bad it can be for your overall well-being, though. Hence, in order to prevent dealing with cell garbage, you need to make sure that the body utilizes autophagy more than apoptosis.

THE THING IS, you cannot completely prevent apoptosis from occurring. It is like telling the liver to stop filtering the blood that passes through your veins. What you can do instead is to make sure that you are controlling the number of times you have to rely on this process.

IMPROVES MUSCLES PERFORMANCE: How?

WHEN YOU WORKOUT, your muscles demand more energy. In order to supply that energy, they turn to autophagy. After all, why not use the energy from damaged cells?

What the body is doing is that it uses a boost of energy from the damaged cells for the muscles.

It is like driving for miles and looking at your gas tank and noticing that you are now out of gas. Fortunately, you have thought ahead and brought along a jerry can with additional fuel, which now lies on the backseat of your car. You stop your vehicle to refuel it, and you practically have an extra supply of gas until you reach the next station.

That is what happens in your body. When you are exercising, you use the energy you have. When you need extra energy, your body turns to its own version of a jerry can: autophagy. The result is a quick boost to help you to exercise longer.

Protecting DNA: How?

According to a scientific report published in Nature by a team of scientists, defecting autophagy in human led to increased DNA damage caused by radiation.

We had always understood how essential autophagy was - and still is - to people, but we never understood just how beneficial it could be on a deep molecular level. The report mentioned above just expands the many functions of autophagy. It shows us how we have been taking for granted an incredibly vital part of our everyday lives.

Humans have evolved over the years. The concept of three meals a day is a recent one. It began during the latter part of the 18th century and stuck with us until now. Before that, we had trained our body to have only the most important nutrients that it could receive. The rest of the time, the body had to find unique methods to cultivate energy and stay fit.

OVER THE YEARS, we have undone everything that we have taught our body to do across a thousand years. We have developed habits that are in contradiction to the very foundations of good health. And, at present, we have noticed how important some of the processes that we have forgotten are, especially on a molecular level.

OUR DNA IS the foundation upon which we function. If there is damage to the structure, then we can see the repercussions of that problem spread out across the body. But our body has a defense mechanism at play. In fact, it has a defense, repair, and maintenance procedures all combined in one process.

THAT PROCESS IS AUTOPHAGY.

*ENHANCES THE IMMUNE SYSTEM: **How?***

OUR IMMUNE SYSTEM is our defense.

THINK about the Lord of the Rings.

IT DOES NOT MATTER if you have watched the movie or not.

. . .

By now, you might be familiar with one particular scene from the movie. It involves a wizard named Gandalf who is shown standing on a bridge. A massive horned creature covered in flames bursts forth from the shadows on the other side of the bridge. As it closes in on Gandalf, the wizard picks up his staff and slams the lower end of it into the bridge shouting, "You shall not pass!"

That's basically your immune system against any kind of foreign object. Trouble is, sometimes, your immune system ends up doing a lot of the heavy lifting, and this can weaken it for a while. In other cases, your immunity may not be enough to fight the invading substances alone.

When the latter happens, doctors prescribe antibiotics to their patients. The main purpose of such medications is to let your body have support when it is fighting whatever bacteria attack you.

In a similar manner, autophagy is like a support mechanism for your immune system. It provides support by removing intracellular pathogens. What this means is that it gets rid of anything that causes disease from the cells of our body. Basically, it flushes the substance or converts it into a source of energy. Not only does it assist the immune system but also helps your body to understand what it is dealing with.

That's like hitting two birds with one stone. Or, two results with just one action.

That is how powerful autophagy can be to your immune system.

. . .

Overall Effects

When you combine the benefits that autophagy provide your body, the overall result is something even more spectacular. The sum of the parts contributes to a wonderful whole.

In the end, you end up having a lot more energy to carry out the work that you want to. You have focus. Your brain functions improves; your memory and thought processes get enhanced. You feel the change as you begin to perform mentally challenging tasks.

Physically, you have better cardiovascular health as well. When you are resting, you need to lower your heart rate. Autophagy ensures that there are no substances blocking the arteries and affecting your heart and the heart rate negatively.

You also have lower levels of stress. When autophagy works on your brain, it helps remove some of the substances causing increased stress. High stress levels pose a whole set of problems of their own. However, when the process starts, you feel more relaxed and calm. You can go through your day without feeling the effects of undue stress.

And let us not forget the markers of aging. Not only does autophagy replace older and damaged cells with younger ones, but it also reduces problems like stress, which contribute towards a more youthful appearance. You feel younger. You act younger. You look younger.

. . .

THOMAS HAWTHORN

But telling you that autophagy reduces stress is like describing the mechanisms of a rocket without giving an introduction to what a rocket is. There is no context, and it is better to understand the basics.

So let's look at stress, shall we?

OXIDATIVE STRESS AND YOUR HORMONES

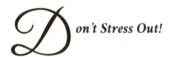 on't Stress Out!

STRESS IS the body's response to any shifts or changes that requires it to provide a reaction or make adjustments. The body responds in one of three ways: physical, mental, or emotional. If you look at the normal functions of human beings, then stress is part of it. In other words, stress is normal.

YOU CAN EXPERIENCE levels of stress due to several factors from the environment. It can be a result of your thought processes or physical changes in your body.

WHEN WE LOOK AT STRESS, we often think that it is a response to negative affects and conditions. That is not always the case. You see, when you encounter positive scenarios like winning the lottery, getting a promotion, birthing your child, or other major situations, that cause positive feelings in you even if it agitates you. Thus, you can say that stress is not always bad.

OUR BODIES ARE TUNED to react to stress. We can handle it. In fact, stress is necessary to keep ourselves motivated, raise our alerts levels, or improve our flight-or-fight responses when we need it.

BUT (AND THERE IS USUALLY A "BUT") ==stress becomes harmful when there is no time for you to relax==. It is like you are constantly on alert without giving yourself any rest.

THE AUTONOMOUS NERVOUS system of our body is designed in such a way that it has a built-in response towards stress. This allows you to manage stressful situations effectively. However, that can only work when you are allowing yourself to rest and recover. Your stress response can become chronic if it is activated for prolonged periods.

LET US USE AN EXAMPLE.

IMAGINE you are riding your bicycle, then you take it through rough terrains. If you do not allow the bicycle to rest or change its tires, then you will not be able to ride it properly in the future.

THIS IS the same with stress. When you are under a stressful situation for long, then you are causing wear and tear on your body. You can notice the effects of the wear both physically and emotionally.

. . .

You might have felt some of the symptoms of stress:

- Exhaustion
- Increased heart rate
- Headaches
- Indigestion
- Aches and pains throughout the body
- Sweaty palms
- Sudden weight gain

All of the factors above are capable of affecting your life drastically.

However, there is another form of stress that is equally harmful to the body: oxidative stress.

Your body constantly feels the effects of oxidative stress. The oxygen in your body separate into single atoms. Typically, an atom is supposed to have a neutron and a proton in the center with electrons in an orbit. These electrons are present in pairs.

Here is something you should know about. Electrons in the atoms always like to be paired. It is how they exist, according to the law of physics.

But in oxidative stress, the oxygen atoms have electrons that are not paired with other electrons.

If they are not paired, then they seek out a pair.

. . .

These unpaired electrons are called free radicals.

The problem with free radicals is that when they are on their quest to seek out electrons to pair with, they often damage the proteins, cells, and DNA that come in their path. This eventually causes numerous problems for the body. Neurodegenerative diseases like Alzheimer's and Parkinson's become common. The body even begins to age faster as the more free radicals accumulate, the more damage they cause.

What exactly causes these free radicals? What leads to their formation?

According to the Huntington's Outreach Project for Education at Stanford University, many of the substances that cause free radicals are found in the food we eat or the things we consume. For example, fried, high-carb or sugar-rich foods, alcohol, and tobacco are some of the typical things that we take, which can bring about the formation of free radicals.

Radicalization of the Body

Rice University in Texas conducted research about the phenomenon to try and understand the various harmful effects of free radicals on the body.[1] What they found was that there's a whole set of reactions that could lead to a rather destructive end.

Let us look at it from the beginning. When free radicals are formed, it creates a chain reaction. When the first free radical is thrown out of a molecule, it disrupts the normal functioning of the latter. The electrons in the molecule, in turn, become free radicals as well. In order to stabilize itself, the molecule takes an electron from another molecule. Now that molecule becomes a free radical. This process continues until, eventually, you see the destructive end that we have mentioned earlier, and the entire cell that hosts these molecules gets damaged. All it took was one electron to set the stage for a chain of reactions.

THE DAMAGE DOES NOT STOP THERE, THOUGH. Your cell membranes can also suffer from free radicals. In some cases, the damaged cells in your body can worsen, mutate, and eventually grow into tumors. If the destruction done by free radicals continues to proceed unchecked, it can change codes in DNA and further lead to other harmful effects. Again, all it took was one free radical to kickstart the chain reaction.

THERE IS MORE damage that can be caused by free radicals, but you get the picture. Some of the effects are short-term and, with the right treatment, you can prevent them from worsening. Others, however, can be life-threatening, especially in the case of tumor formation. Still, the situation can only get worse (as if it hasn't gotten bad already).

Flame On! Inflammation Makes a Comeback

WHEN YOU HAVE high stress levels for long periods, then your body turns to other means of stress management.

IT TURNS to inflammation for help.

YES, that is the wrong move.

. . .

THEN YOU HAVE a host of other problems that take over the body. You have stress and inflammation going hand-in-hand doing damage to your body, both in the short-term and over a longer course of time.

YOU HAVE short-term effects like sleep deprivation, damage to your gut, and headaches. Then you have the long-term effects such as slow weight gain, bone damage and skin problems.

SOME OF THE above problems lead to further damage. A good night's sleep is how the body powers up its immune system and gives your brain a well-deserved rest. Without it, your immune system gets compromised and you end might just end up receiving a high dose of depression.

BEFORE YOU KNOW IT, your body is dealing with multiple problems. You have oxidized stress going about wreaking havoc. You have symptoms of the oxidized stress creating more problems. Then you have the body trying to manage the problem by using a process that should be supposed to help, but only leads to more problems.

THINGS ARE NOT LOOKING good for the body.

IF THINGS CONTINUE, then you are looking at a host of problems and wondering just what you should be taking care of first.

THE REASON why these problems prevail is because we haven't exactly provided our body with any alternatives. It is like handing over a roadmap with just one road leading from the point of origin to the destination.

But what if we had the power to provide the body an alternate course of action? What if we could let the body know that it does not have to depend in inflammation to solve its problems?

Surely that would make the work for your body a whole lot easier wouldn't it?

Thankfully, this entire book is focused on a process which could very well be the alternative course of action that the body is looking for.

Autophagy vs. Oxidized Stress

Think about it.

If autophagy had begun working its magic during the oxidized stress phase, then you can prevent any further problems from developing. In fact, let us assume that we have free radicals going around damaging cells in the body.

What should be the solution there? What should be done to these damaged cells so that they in turn cannot cause further harm?

. . .

I AM sure at this point, you might have already guessed the answer and figured out what should happen to those cells.

YOU ARE RIGHT. Bring in autophagy and let it recycle these cells. After all, they are not going to be useful anymore and if they continue to remain unchecked, they are only going to cause more problems. Let us simply nip the problem at the bud.

OR IN THIS CASE, nip it at the cellular level.

LET us look at this from another viewpoint. Let us assume that the problem has proceeded into a pretty dangerous area. Inflammation is about to take place and the body does not have any options left on the table.

NOW, we do not have to wait for the situation to get worse. If you can introduce intermittent fasting and autophagy at this point, then we can still make sure that we can manage the situation without further damage.

AND THAT MAKES autophagy not just useful, but dynamic as well. We do not have to feel that we are too late to do anything to reverse the damage caused. In many cases, we can introduce autophagy and try to minimize the harmful effects of whatever process is creating trouble in our body.

BUT WE HAVE BEEN LOOKING at the effects of what a poor diet can cause to the body. We haven't actually focused on the food itself.

. . .

WHAT IF I told you that some doctors believe that the calorie-in-calorie-out method might very well have been a bigger disaster than World War 2?

SURPRISED? Shocked? Well, don't be because we are about to explore more about it.

A MATTER OF BELIEF: THE COLOSSAL FAILURE OF THE CALORIE IN, CALORIE OUT MODEL AND THE AMERICAN DIET SYSTEM

Doctors are given very little information about leading a healthy lifestyle. However, they are well-versed in the prescription of drugs.

In recent years, this trend of simply relying on prescriptions is changing. More and more discoveries are made about leading healthy lifestyles, adopting a nutritious and well-balanced diet, and taking advantage of exercises and workout routines to develop the body.

YOU SEE, if everyone told you that all you need to do is be cautious about the food you eat and simply head over to the gym or indulge in activities to lead a better lifestyle, then who is going to consume all the prescription drugs manufactured by pharmaceuticals?

THAT DOES NOT MEAN that there is an evil corporation about to take over the world and right at the top is a lunatic cackling in glee with a maniacal laughter.

. . .

WHAT I MEAN IS that too often, doctors forget to give long-term recommendations. When you start digging deeper into how a healthy diet makes positive contributions to our health, you start uncovering useful tips, habits, and choices. If pharmaceuticals spend more time on such endeavors, they could provide a permanent solution to all our problems within a single sheet of paper.

THINK OF THIS STATISTIC: according to NHS England, lifestyle related diseases such as heart diseases and diabetes is a 16 billion pound industry! That is a lot of money to be spent on problems that you can basically manage with the right dietary advice and a careful application of fitness into the daily routine of the people.

HOWEVER, that would mean a loss of nearly 16 billion pounds for the medical industry.

LET us look at another situation. Rather, let us examine a certain belief that was held true for so long that people's lives were affected by it.

THE CALORIE THEORY OF OBESITY.

THIS THEORY MIGHT JUST BE a blot in the history of medicine. It has been known as one of the most colossal failures in medical history. This belief system has led to the deaths of many people who went to adopt a method that had no real benefit in their lives.

HOW DID IT HAPPEN?

. . .

THE CALORIE THEORY of obesity is based on a gross misunderstanding of the equation for energy balance.

HERE IS the gist of the equation.

THE AMOUNT of body fat gained = the number of calories taken in − the number of calories exhausted (or left the body).

THAT EQUATION SOUNDS SIMPLY DOESN'T it?

IN FACT, most people could take a quick glance at the equation and say, "Well, all we need to do now is to balance out the calories we took in by working out and spending those calories."
Or.
"Perhaps I could lower the calories I take. That would mean that I can still exercise less and be able to balance out the fat I consume. Easy peasy!"

So, what does all this man?

WELL, let us use an example to highlight this point. Calories that amount to 3,500 are equal to about a pound of fat. According to the calorie in, calorie out method, if you have about 500 calories less every day compared to the amount of calories that you burn, then by the end of the week, you have lost about 3,500 calories (500 calories per day x 7 days).

YOU HAVE ACTUALLY LOST one pound of fat at the end of the week!

. . .

SIMPLE, isn't it?

WHAT ARE WE WAITING FOR? Let's just get started on this rather ingenious method.

HOWEVER, it is a major problem if you are only focusing on the number of calories you consume and the number of calories you spend. It is an extremely simplified way of thinking and it does not always work in the way that you think.

IF YOUR ONLY focus is on calories, and you neglect to include the metabolic effects of those calories, then you are throwing out important factors that lead to weight gain.

THE FIRST LAW of thermodynamics reminds us that energy cannot be created or destroyed. It simply exists. It can change form. But it cannot be simply extinguished from this world.

WHEN THE ENERGY gained by the body is more than the energy leaving the body, then that excess energy gets stored as fat. So far, so good. We all know this.

So, the obvious conclusion to the above train of thought is this: take in more calories, gain more weight. The logic is irrefutable. It is based on physics.

. . .

However, that is all it does.

It states the obvious.

It does not explain anything else.

If you take in calories, you gain weight. But why? Why are you gaining weight?

Let me explain with another example.

Let us assume that you are about to enter a restaurant but it is very crowded. A few of the diners exit the restaurant.

You stop them ask them why the restaurant is packed tonight. They respond by saying, "well that is because more people have entered the restaurant than people who have exited."

What does that even mean?!

That is not the answer you were looking for. You want to know the reason behind the crowd. Is there a popular dish on the menu? Is there a discount? Are they giving out free wine? What is it?

It is the same with obesity. Simply saying that calorie intake makes you fat does not explain anything.

You need more answers to figure out the problem. Why are people consuming more calories?

. . .

Has it got something to with the hormones? Is it the habits that the person has formed over the years? Is it a behavioral problem?

Additionally, people who believe in the calorie in and calorie out method are of the opinion that all calories are the same. It is the only way they can come to the conclusion that by simply working out or consuming less calories, you can lose a certain amount of fat by the end of the week.

But the reality is much more complex. Different sources of fats function in different ways.

Let us examine the above point with a few examples.

100 Calories of Fructose

When you consume fructose, it is taken to the liver where is converted to glycogen. The thing is, liver already has a certain amount of glycogen. Any excess is either taken to other fat deposits in the body or accumulates in the liver, causing more harm to it.

But the thing about fructose is that the body does not recognize it or treat it the same way that it treats other sugars like glucose.

Fructose does not lower insulin levels in the body. This means that your body continues to remain hungry and you end up eating more. That results in weight gain.

. . .

Glucose on the other hand can lower insulin levels, so you are not constantly feeling hungry.

100 Calories of Protein

Firstly, part of the protein that you consume is actually spend on digesting it. Secondly, protein makes you full. Thirdly, proteins are used to build muscles!

100 Calories of Fructose vs. 100 Calories of Protein

If you were taking into consideration only the calorie count, then you might have ignored what you have consumed.

To people who believe in the calorie in and calorie out method, they might think that as they have consumed about 100 calories, they have to lose 100 calories.

But what if it was proteins that they consumed? They are practically trying to remove a good source of energy for the body.

And that's where the problem lies.

If calorie in and calorie out took into consideration the diet that people consume, then we might be looking at the equation like this:
 The amount of body fat gained = the number of calories taken in − the number of calories exhausted (or left the body)

. . .

THAT BASICALLY CHANGES the entire perspective of the equation. Now you are going to be more cautious about how you measure calories. You might think, "Wait, what am I eating? What kind of calories am I consuming? Perhaps I should look at my daily diet."

HOWEVER, you are never told the truth about calorie in and calorie out. In fact, many people continue to believe in the equation because their doctor or health practitioner might have explained it to them, without highlighting anything about the food they eat or the type of calories they consume.

IF DOCTORS GAVE out really specific instructions on the type of food that someone should eat in order to maintain their health and lose weight, then they won't have to prescribe any medicines.

HOW ARE those who manufacture those medicines going to get money?

ADDITIONALLY, how are food manufacturers going to get money?

WAIT. How did the food industry get into this equation.

LET ME TELL YOU WHY.

ARE YOU A FOODIE?

. . .

THINK about some of the most popular foods consumed by Americans.

HOT DOGS. Hamburgers. Potato Chips. Soda.

ALL OF THESE foods are made using compounds created by corn. Sounds rather unbelievable right?

THAT'S why we have the science to back us up. So, let us try looking at each food and seeing how they are manufactured using corn.

MOST OF THE sodas and drinks that you consume (think Gatorade, Coca-Cola, Monster, etc.) contain corn syrup.

HAMBURGERS, hot dogs and the fried chickens that you get at your favorite fast food joint use meat from animals that have been fed corn. Why corn? Because a diet that's based on corn means that the animals take less time to fatten. This way, they can meet the growing demands of the popular food in the market.

POTATO CHIPS. Though the entire emphasis is on the potato, a lot of your favorite snacks are made using enriched corn meal. This is important to add flavor into the chips and minimize the use of potatoes (potatoes are rather expensive, after all).

IN MANY WAYS, corn is big industry. In fact, it has been estimated that biotech products manufactured using corn amounted to over $125 billion in the year 2012.

AUTOPHAGY

. . .

THAT'S JUST the biotech industry. Wait till we start including every other product that uses corn and you might just get an idea how profitable corn manufacturing can just be.

IT IS for this reason that the corn industry (among other food industries) aim to dissuade people from turning to healthier sources of food.

JUST HEAD over to your nearest supermarket. If you look at the shelves, then you will realize that nearly 3 out of 4 products are made using corn or compounds of corn.

THIS MEANS that no matter what choice you make regarding your diet, you might just end up consuming corn. Additionally, most of the big food industries have taken on another method to combat the awareness of healthy food diets.

THE WAY they do this is by slapping labels such as "low-carb" on many of their products.

THAT LABEL DEFINITELY SOUNDS TEMPTING. After all, if the product is low-carb, it is definitely going to be safe to consume. Here is the reality. It does sound tempting to consume such items, but the bottom line is that they do not provide you with any real benefit.

THIS IS because there is no nutritional guideline that is set up to explain just what low-carb means. It is entirely up to the manufacturer to decide what they feel constitutes a low amount of carbs in their food.

And the worst part is that low-carb foods are actually priced more than regular foods. The idea that people might spend more in the hopes that they can enjoy the food that they want without sacrificing the health is exactly what the food manufacturers want.

But if a product says low-carb, then it surely must have a decrease in the amount of carbs. It should definitely be a healthier option than trying out other options. Right?

Well, it depends on what you mean by healthy and how you gauge the level of benefits provided to you by the product.

Let us look at an example. If you have taken a good that has the label "low-carb," you might be surprised to find out that the carb levels are actually seven to eight times higher than the ones mentioned on the label.

That definitely does not sound right. Why isn't the FDA doing anything? Where is the outrage?

This is where guidelines are important. If there are established guidelines that dictate the way carbs are supposed to be mentioned on packaging, then food manufacturers cannot simply place a label with any number of calories.

. . .

However, that is not the case because those guidelines are practically non-existent. It is entirely up to the manufacturer to decide what they think is low-carb to them.

When you consume low-carb foods, you are inadvertently causing harm in your body. For one, you haven't changed your diet. You are feeding it the same amount of substances that you had been feeding it earlier.

This means that you are causing the same reactions to occur in the body.

Take for example insulin.

Inside Insulin

If low-carb foods are supposed to be helpful, then biologically, they are supposed to lower your insulin levels. This means that your hunger levels are supposed to dissipate. But try eating low-carb chips next time and see if it has any effect on your hunger levels. Many people end up consuming multiple packets of low-carb chips under the belief that they are not doing the body any harm. They feel hungry after one packet and they go for another. Pretty soon, they have just consumed multiple packets.

Let us look at another substance: fructose.

. . .

As we had seen before, many of the products on the supermarket shelf consist of compounds made with corn. One of those compounds is corn syrup. Products made with this substance have high degree of fructose. Here is a fact about fructose, though: it gets absorbed slowly. This means that they might just end up not getting absorbed in the intestine and continue on towards the colon. When this happens, it starts getting fermented in the colon. This causes bloating and diarrhea. You are eventually left with a condition called Irritable Bowel Syndrome or IBS.

You can tell that you are in for a whole lot of unpleasantness when you have a syndrome with the word "irritable" and "bowel" in it.

Let's not delay the inevitable and look at what this syndrome can do to your body.

- You are going to experience abdominal pain and cramping. Typically, the pain should reduce with your bowel movement. However, there is no guarantee of that happening.
- You are going to experience diarrhea and constipation in alternative sequences. This means you are going to experience one at one time and then the other at a different time. All while still enduring your abdominal pain. Oh, yeah, it is about to get worse.
- You are going to experience an increase in gas production in the intestines. And that just leads to more embarrassing situations we do not want to explain in detail.

AUTOPHAGY

Suffice it to say, the condition is painful, uncomfortable, and embarrassing. And it is all simply because you have increased the dosage of fructose.

Surprisingly, you might not even be aware that some of the products you consume have fructose in them. Because - let me hit you with another fact - even ==certain fruits and honey have fructose in them.==

Let me be clear; you need fructose in small quantities. The amount you consume from fruits and in small doses, honey, is useful for you. This is true when you are working out or exercising regularly.

The problem is with the products in the supermarket. They are made to have high levels of fructose. This is done in order to bring out the flavor in the products. When your body receives such high doses of sugar, it becomes hooked. It is like taking drugs. Your body gets a "feel good" moment that only lasts for a short while until the next quick fix.

In fact, according to the US National Library of Medicine National Institutes of Health, high fructose content leads to impairment in the dopamine production in your body. This means that you might just feel good about taking in fructose, even though your body might not want it. Your dependency grows and food manufacturers keep on getting richer.

For this reason, manufacturers do not go out of their way to try and explain what is included in their products. They are not bound by the rules that cigarette companies need to follow. When any product contains tobacco, to be specific, a warning label must be placed on it.

Unfortunately, food companies do not have to put on such labels. If they did, then people might just become more aware of what they are eating.

Trick or Treat: **How Food Manufacturers Trick Customers into Eating Their Treats**

Let us examine a myth.

The Myth

Ingredients listed on food products are designed to be informative. They are accurate. They tell the complete picture of what the customer can expect from the product and what they are about to consume.

The Reality

Not even close to the myth that we just examined. The reality is that the listed ingredients are created by food manufacturers to trick consumers and into having a certain perception about the food. In other words, the manufacturers want people believing that the products are healthier.

However, aren't there certain requirements that these manufacturers have to follow? Can they blatantly lie about what they include in the foods they create?

. . .

IN MANY CASES, they don't lie. But that does not mean that they are giving you the complete picture.

HERE ARE some ways that the nutrition facts that you find on products are deceiving.

- A common trick employed (and quite frankly, still practiced) is to distribute the sugars among different ingredients in the food. This way, they do not have to list the sugar based ingredients on the top of the list. When you read the label, you might notice a sugar compound in the beginning, followed by other ingredients. The sugar-based ingredient on the top has a low sugar level. You automatically believe that the product you are going to consume has low levels of carbs, not knowing that the remaining sugar-based ingredients are at the bottom. For example, a manufacturer may use different sources of sugar such as high-fructose corn syrup, sucrose, brown sugar, powdered sugar and other sugar and place them into different ingredients. Now, all they have to do is show the names of the ingredients, not the names of the sugar. If they can keep the levels of these sugar-based ingredients low, then they can list ALL of them at the bottom. All the non-sugar based components goes on top. Voila! You now have a healthy product with low sugar content. Pretty cunning, isn't it?
- Ready for trick number two? In the second trick, the manufacturers cover the list with small amounts of ingredients that have really fancy names. You might often spot these kinds of names in personal care or cosmetic products that often go by the claim of offering you something "herbal" when in reality, there are no trace amounts of herbs inside these products. When it comes to food, manufacturers hide the real ingredients with healthy

sounding fruits, berries, and nuts. These items are available in trace amounts, but that does not stop the labels from listing them. Having an item that says "spirulina" does not mean anything. It is only available in small amounts and won't contribute to any health benefit at all. In fact, it is as good as not consuming the ingredient at all. However, the trick is to show customers that there are healthy ingredients inside the food. It is not a matter of how much. It is a matter of whether there is or not.

- We now come to the third trick. This time, manufacturers use the art of camouflage. In this method the ingredients are listed using another name, something that is related to their chemical composition or the way scientists label them. When you look at the label and see the term maltodextrin, you won't think twice about it. It could mean something that is extracted from fruits or nuts. But here is the kicker. Maltodextrin is nothing but another name for sugar. What about disaccharides? It sounds innocent enough, but nope - that is sugar again. Sodium nitrite? That's not sugar. However, sodium nitrate has been known to contribute towards the formation of various cancer types include pancreatic and colon cancer.

WITH JUST A FEW WORDS, the entire content of a product changes. When you look at these products, you are completely unaware of what is inside them. This is because nobody knows what maltodextrin is.

MANUFACTURERS EXPECT the customer to remain ignorant. It is how they can continue to label the products in a manner that fits them.

. . .

HAVE you come across products that have the word "Light" on them? They have a wonderful color to match their theme, preferably green or light yellow. This is done to give off the look of a product that has natural ingredients. However, many products that have "Light" on them might reduce fat or calories by removing certain ingredients. Instead, they sometimes add in sugar.

IT IS up to you to become aware of what you are about to eat. You need to make sure that you are not falling prey to either false labelling or brand reputation. For example, Quaker oats is a rather popular product in supermarkets. In fact, when the term "healthy breakfast" appears, you can be sure that there is someone out there considering buying a Quaker oat product. The thing is, the person who is on the Quaker logo is not the founder of the brand. In fact, everything about the brand is designed to make it seem as though it is healthy (even the font type). Most people look at the logo and immediately make a purchase of the product. They do not even check the ingredients on the back. After all, it is Quakers, right? They are reputed! There is no need to mistrust them! Your prudence is your best friend. Of course, that does not mean that there is an evil corporation out to get you. Everything that manufacturers do is to stay ahead of the competition and ensure that their products sell. Sometimes, they may not always make the right decisions when it comes to marketing.

ONLY YOU ARE capable of making the right judgement.

AUTOPHAGY AND INSULIN

The term 'cancer' is a name given to a collection of diseases. Different types of cancer affect different parts of the body. But they have the same process: various cells in the body begin to divide uncontrollably. These cells then spread around to affect nearby tissues.

CANCER CAN BEGIN in any part of the body. Usually, human cells tend to develop and divide to create new cells whenever the body requires them. When cells become damaged or when they age, the next step in their life is death. When these cells die, newer cells replace them.

THIS WAY, your body keeps you healthy and ensures that there is no disruption in any function in the body.

WHEN YOUR BODY is affected by cancer, the disease affects your body's ability to create new cells. As more cells start getting damaged or old and they continue to survive instead of being replaced, then your body starts producing new cells when it is not required (after all, the older cells have to be removed in order to introduce new cells in the body, else there will be an excess of cells). These extra cells end up dividing without control and may form harmful growths called tumors.

IN MANY FORMS OF CANCER, you might notice the formation of solid tissues. However, in other forms of cancer such as leukemia, there is an absence of any solid tissue. Regardless of the presence of these tissues, there is no form of cancer that is worse than the other. Each have their own way of destroying the body and each type of cancer should be given complete attention.

TUMORS THAT ARE cancerous are typically malignant. What this means is that they can continue spreading and end up affecting nearby tissues as well. In many instances, while the tumor grows, some of the cells can separate from the main mass and travel to other places in the body. Eventually, they form new tumors.

THE NEW TUMORS are typically benign. What this means is that the new tumors don't spread or attack tissues close to them. Additionally, when you remove benign tumors from your body, they do not grow back. The same may not apply to malignant tumor, because there are chances that these tumors can grow back even if you remove them.

How Does Cancer Harm the Body?

THERE ARE MORE than 100 types of cancer. Most types are named after the area of the body where they spread. For example, brain cancer begins in the brain and lung cancer starts with the cells in the lungs.

. . .

However, cancers are typically classified into five main types.

Sarcoma

Sarcomas is the type of cancer that forms in the bones and soft tissues. There are many types of soft tissues that are in the body. You have muscle fat, lymph vessels, blood vessels, and even fibrous tissues.

Carcinoma

These cancers begin in the cells or tissues that line the internal organs. These are the most common types of cancer.

Leukemia

Leukemia is a cancer that forms in the bone marrow or blood. One of the things to remember about this cancer is that they do not have a solid mass. Rather, they begin to spread abnormal white blood cells in the blood and bone marrow. Because of this, the normal blood cells get outnumbered and may not be able to move around the body freely. When the level of normal blood cells becomes too low, then it becomes difficult for the body to divert oxygen to various tissues in the body, fight infections, or even control bleeding.

Lymphoma

. . .

AUTOPHAGY

LYMPHOMA TYPE of cancer that affects the immune system or begins in the immune system. This cancer begins in the lymphocytes, which are the while blood cells responsible for fighting diseases. This means that the body's ability to fight diseases becomes severely hampered.

CENTRAL NERVOUS SYSTEM Cancers

THESE BEGIN in the spinal cord or in the brain.

Each of the above forms of cancer have their own set of symptoms and side effects. They cause harm in their own way.

Autophagy and Cancer

CERTAIN CANCERS TRY and resist against treatments such as radiotherapy or chemotherapy because they use various methods or techniques for survival.

BUT RECENTLY, scientists have discovered a way of getting through one of cancer's defense mechanisms.

AT THIS POINT, I don't need to tell you what that way is.

WE KNOW that when autophagy is triggered, cells break down the compounds that are useless or capable of causing more harm to the body and recycle the material as energy. Because of this, autophagy creates complications for cancer cells. It helps your body to try and destroy them or in many cases, stop the progression of cancer.

. . .

67

MOST OF THE research has been conducted on mice. However, the thing to remember is that the behavioral and biological makeup of mice closely resemble those of humans. That is usually why you notice scientists often using mice for their research. They know that if their theories prove right on the rodents, then they can move further and advance their studies. They could even move on to human trials.

HAVING SAID THAT, let us move on back to autophagy. One of the things that happens when autophagy takes over is that it can constrain the creation of tumor by managing the damage that DNA receives due to various processes in the body. Furthermore, we have already seen how autophagy can control oxidative stress. When you combine the effects of the regulation of damaged DNA and the reduction of oxidative stress, then you are lowering your chances of creating tumorous cells in your body. Thus, the medical community often say that targeting autophagy is an efficient cancer therapy method.

SO FAR, we have seen successes only in clinical trials. But scientists believe that it won't be long before they are able to start recommending it to people.

WE HAVE NOW ESTABLISHED what an important role autophagy plays in the management of cancer. That does not mean you can simply jump into a fasting process and try activating autophagy. You need to understand that you might have to take certain precautions first.

LET US LOOK INTO THAT.

BEING CAUTIOUS: PRECAUTIONS TO TAKE REGARDING AUTOPHAGY AND FASTING

Let's get this out of the way; you do not have to activate autophagy every day. Many people become obsessed with making sure that their body gets as much benefits as possible from autophagy. They end up trying to encourage it to happen every day.

I am not saying that having autophagy work for you everyday is bad. However, you need to make sure that you understand what your goals are.

There are three main ways to induce autophagy.

Fasting

Typically, you have to work on intermittent fasting to ensure that you start the autophagy process properly. There are many types of intermittent fasting options that you can take advantage of and that can be perfect for you. Once again, think about what you are trying to achieve through fasting and then you might have a clear picture of how you would like to fast.

Ketogenic Diet

THE BENEFIT of the keto diet is that it is a high-fat and low-carb diet. Its main purpose is to flush out the bad fats in your body gained from sugar and carbs. Then, it turns your body's attention to using the good fats that it receives from specific diets.

EXERCISE

EXERCISE IS KNOWN to boost the autophagy process when you combine it with fasting and keto diet. Additionally, working on your body makes you feel healthier and enhances your muscles even more.

So let us try and understand the best way to begin the intermittent fasting process and eventually, get your autophagy into motion.

THE FASTING *and the Furious*

THERE ARE several ways you can perform intermittent fasting. These ways are built to cater to a specific requirement or lifestyle. This means that you can adopt any of the fasting methods mentioned below to suit your needs.

Let us look at some of the most popular methods of fasting right now.

. . .

The 16/8 Method

In this method, you do not consume breakfast. Rather you place your period of eating anywhere between 1pm to 9pm (an 8-hour window). When eating, you will only be focused on having a keto diet. Once you have finished your meal, your next step would be to fast for 16 hours.

Eat-Stop-Eat

This is an extreme method of fasting and people usually do it once a week. In this method, you fast for a period of 24 hours. The way to do this is by not eating dinner one day and refusing to eat until dinner time the next day. People often prepare themselves before they try out the eat-stop-eat method.

The 5:2 Diet

In this method, you consume about 500 to 600 calories on two days of the week. On the remaining days, you can continue to eat normally. However, with the recent understanding of how calorie in and calorie out is not the way to look at your food, this method might not be suitable for you, especially if you are planning to lose weight.

One Meal a Day (OMAD)

. . .

Let us now look at the most popular type of intermittent fasting: the OMAD. In this method, you only make sure that you eat only once during the day. The OMAD consists of high-fat and low-carb diet.

When you understand the mechanics of fasting, then you can easily find out a routine that works for you and helps you realize the goal you have set forth for yourself. However, choosing the right method of fasting is just the beginning.

What to Eat

When you are fasting, the best diet to adopt is the keto diet. The reason is that this diet ensures that you receive the substances that are positive for your body and help you during the fasting period. You also end up feeling good about your progress and begin to notice positive changes within yourself.

What to Drink

Ideally, you are going to avoid sugary drinks. You are going to restrict yourself to drinking the below fluids:

- Sparkling water
- Mineral water
- Plain black coffee
- Plain tea

There are other liquids that you can take, but we will be discussing them further in the book.

How to Exercise

. . .

WHEN YOU EXERCISE during your fasting period, make sure that you restrict yourself to workouts or routines that are under 60 minutes. This not only allows you to take advantage of the fasting, but makes certain that you do not add too much stress on your body. After all, you are supposed to have a fast that is as comfortable as possible.

EAT WELL: FOODS THAT BOOST AUTOPHAGY

What we know so far is that autophagy is the process of either flushing out or recycling old or damaged cells. It occurs during fasting or starvation; however, we prefer to start it during fasting rather than starvation. It is beneficial to us in many ways.

WE ALSO KNOW by now that ketosis is the state where the body produces high ketones and ensures that these ketones are utilized as much as possible.

Hone Your Ketone

WHEN YOU DO NOT HAVE enough sugar in the body, mainly in the form of glucose, then your body uses other forms of fuel. The glycogen, blood sugar, and insulin levels are lowered at this point. The body then starts looking for alternate sources of fuel. In this case, it is looking for fat.

. . .

THIS PROCESS usually happens when you enter a state of fasting. At this point, you have to ensure that you feed the body fats from keto diet. And when the body begins consuming fats for energy, another process called beta-oxidation takes over. During this process, ketones are produced for as fuel for the body and brain. Your body enters into a state of ketosis.

IN OTHER WORDS, ketones are food fuel, the one you should be consuming more.

NOW THAT WE understand autophagy and ketosis, it is time to see why they go hand-in-hand, as though they are partners in a buddy cop movie.

YOU SEE, when autophagy activates, then it gets rid of the old cells in the body. Basically, all the bad stuff in your body is slowly getting recycled as energy. At this point, it is time for you to introduce your body to healthy substances. More specifically, you need to provide a healthy source of energy to your body. Autophagy alone cannot be a source of energy.

IF YOU GO BACK to a high-carb diet, then all the efforts you have out into your diet up until now is practically gone to waste. This is why your next step is to focus on bringing in positive sources of energy. And what better way than introducing your body to ketosis?

THINK OF IT LIKE THIS: out goes bad cells, and in comes good fats and energy.

. . .

You might ask at this point: now that I know about taking in good energy, just what do I need to eat or consume during my intermittent fasting period?

There are a lot of foods that encourage the process of autophagy.

Let us look at some of them.

- Make sure that you try to include spices that boost autophagy and are considered as "autophagy-friendly." The most popular spices that you can use are ginger, cumin, and ginseng.
- Include foods that are high in resveratrol, which is a compound that occurs naturally and is found in a number of fruits. Resveratrol itself belongs to another family of compounds called polyphenolic compounds or polyphenols for short. These compounds act as antioxidants. Some of the foods that are rich in resveratrol are mulberries, pomegranate, raspberries, and blueberries.
- See if you can include organ meats into your diet. Organ meats, as the name implies, refer to the organs of animals that are consumed for food. Typically, you might notice parts such as liver, tongue, and kidneys as part of the menu where they serve organ meats. You might obviously think that organ meat sounds like a rather strange addition to this list. However, consuming the meat provides your body with numerous nutritional benefits. To begin with, organ meat consist of essential components such as vitamin B12 and folate. Additionally, you can extract all sorts of minerals from them such as magnesium, iron, zinc, and selenium. Most importantly however, they are rich in proteins. When

you are fasting, you need to make sure that you consume enough protein. This helps you build your muscles, which becomes even more important when you are working out or exercising during your fast.

- **Eggs.** Ever since man discovered them, they have been part of our diets and our cuisines. With eggs, you get a complete nutrient profile. In fact, the egg yolk and egg white separately provide you with so many benefits that they should be an ideal part of your diet. One of the things that makes eggs quite popular is the fact that they are an inexpensive source of protein. More than 50% of the protein of the egg is found in the white. The egg white also contains vitamin B2. Egg yolks on the other hand contain vitamins A, D, E, and K. You can have the egg by itself in many ways, or by adding it as an ingredient in another food. Either way, you should make sure that an egg is part of your diet.

I HAVE COVERED MUCH MORE about ketogenic autophagy, the foods that you can eat during your fasting period and, of course, some incredibly delicious recipes for you to adopt for your keto diet. You can find all that and more in my book *Ketogenic Autophagy: Combine the Keto Diet & Nobel Prize Winning Science to Look and Feel Younger, Lose Weight, and Extend Your Life + 28 Day OMAD Meal Plan.*

FOR NOW, we are going to start looking at the autophagy lifestyle and discuss just how you can bring about better health, better diet, and even better vitality among other benefits into your life.

AUTOPHAGY LIFESTYLE: HOW TO INCORPORATE FASTING INTO YOUR DAILY LIFE

*I*deally, you should be aiming to fast without trying to consume any macronutrients. However, it is always good to know that there are certain macros that can start autophagy. This helps you plan your diet and fast much better.

But the question is: What macros are useful? What should you be focusing on?

Here is the first thing that you should know. If your goal is to start autophagy and when you are eating, then you should make sure that you include some form of mealtime restrictions. You can try fasting for about 20 hours, for instance, and then eat roughly 40% to 50% of the amount of energy you spend on a daily basis.

When you are taking in macros, you should ensure that they follow the guidelines below:

- Low in carbohydrates
- Have medium protein content

You should also think about adding food with fats (as discussed in my book *Ketogenic Autophagy*).

So, ideally, your food should have these ratios:

- 10% carbs
- 20% protein
- 25% to 30% fat
- 50% caloric deficit

This ensures that you have the right amount of macros available to you, and you do not have to stop the autophagy process at any point in time. At the same time, you are taking in low carbs.

Though whenever I mention low carbs to people, one of the common questions that I get asked is: What is the difference between a low-carb and a keto diet?

One may look at both forms of diet and think that they are both going to generate the same results. So, it does not matter if you switch one diet for the other.

The reason why people think that they are the same is that both low-carb and keto diets are aimed at reducing and, in some cases, removing the body's dependency on carbohydrates. When examined closely, you may spot differences, especially in the way that they affect your health.

To understand what we mean by that, let us try to look at each form of diet.

Low-Carb Diet

Here is a surprising fact. According to Government Dietary Guidelines for Americans, carbohydrates take up to 65% of your daily food intake.

That is a big percentage. And not a good one.

Here is another fact: There are no guidelines to tell you exactly what low-carb diet means. There are no measurements to quantify the amount of carbohydrates that make up this plan. In truth, we have noticed how this provides an excuse for manufacturers to add the term "low carb" on their labels. In the same way, a low-carb diet can mean anything. Someone can tell you that they have the best recommendations for a low-carb diet and you may not be able to say anything against it because it might very well be true.

Keto Diet

While the rules of a low-carb diet are not exactly concrete, keto diet works with some rules on how you approach your low-carb situation.

You need to enter a state, which is known as ketosis (a term that we have already understood earlier).

IN ORDER for you to go into ketosis state, you need to make sure that you have a calorie count of less than 50 grams a day. By letting you know just how much calories you can consume, you are given a guideline. You can understand what you can include in your diet and what you should avoid.

OF COURSE, as we have said in previous chapters, calories are not everything. However, when you have a certain number to aim for, you can then use that as a benchmark to decide on what you are going to eat. With that, you can make sure that you are consuming the right amount of nutrients from the right source. A keto diet can make it easier for you to focus on losing weight while keeping you full.

A STUDY WAS ONCE CONDUCTED on two groups of people. One group was given a keto diet with just 4% of carbs. The other group was given a low-carb diet with about 25% carbs. The result? The people of the keto diet saw better. They experienced the following:

- They felt less hungry than the individuals who were on a low-carb diet.
- They lost more weight.
- They ate fewer calories than the people on the low-carb diet!

A KETO DIET works its magic in many ways. If you want to lose weight or simply change your lifestyle, then you are looking at a keto diet to help you out.

. . .

Nevertheless, is it all about having less calories? Are there more benefits that you can take away from a keto diet? Of course, there is.

Let us examine a few of them.

- Keto provides your body with more physical and mental energy to handle a lot of activities, from workouts to tasks at the office to just enjoying time with your family and friends. The reason for this is of course the fuel you have in the form of ketones; they are much more efficient than using other sources of fuel such as glucose. Additionally, your brain has something called the blood-brain barrier. What this barrier does is keep as many of the harmful materials from entering the brain as possible. In other words, substances that are too large cannot pass through this barrier and enter the brian. Ketones on the other hand are able to bypass this barrier. This means your brain can also enjoy some of the good energy that the rest of the body receives. You become more focused. Your stress levels drops. You have better functionality of your brain.
- Ketosis may provide your body with protection against neurodegenerative diseases. That much is obvious because we have seen why it does so in an earlier chapter. But here is the kicker: it gives you a long-term protection against such diseases. This is not something you can gain from a low-carb diet. One of the reasons why the keto diet was created was so that it could help people with epilepsy avoid periods of seizures. In fact, for many years, neurologists have shown that the keto diet has been effective in people who are resistant to drugs that reduce epilepsy.
- Ketones are also known to act as antioxidants. This helps

your brain shield itself from oxidative stress and from damages caused by stress.

WHEN YOU COMBINE the process of ketosis with autophagy, then we are looking at a host of benefits that help you live a long life that is devoid of numerous health complications.

SO NOW THAT we have understood just how a keto diet is useful, what exactly are the various fasting types that we can make use of to activate ketosis and autophagy?

LET me help you with that.

BEFORE I PROCEED, I must tell you that these fasting techniques are not the ones I had mentioned earlier. Sure, those fasting techniques are some of the most popular ones, but in order to activate ketosis and take full advantage of autophagy, here are the techniques that you should be following:

OMAD (ONE MEAL a Day)
A time-restricted feeding basically means that you are going to eat during a specific period of the day. During the remaining hours, you are going to fast. OMAD is a type of fasting that focuses on time-restricted eating. OMAD simply means "One Meal a Day" and the name says it all; you are going to have just one meal a day. One really healthy, filling and delicious meal a day.

. . .

The name does sounds rather exotic. But it is a rather simple process that forces you in an OMAD plan, you follow a 23/1 fasting routine. You fast for 23 hours and then you have 1 hour to eat your food.

Alternatively, it can also be a 22/2 fasting routine. Here, you fast for 22 hours and then you take 2 hours to slowly eat your food. Eating food has numerous benefits as I have discussed in my book Ketogenic Autophagy.

But back to OMAD. Typically, people wait until dinnertime to break their fast. They use one of the many keto recipes to prepare a filling and healthy meal for themselves. The end result is that OMAD is an extreme way of doing intermittent fasting.

Protein Fasting

When you think about it, fasting is simply a pattern of eating.
You hold out on eating throughout the day and keep one time (or a few specific times, depending on what kind of fast you are holding) to have a meal that is filled with a certain type of substance (example: fat, proteins, etc.)

In many fasting techniques, people use only water. In other techniques, people use a combination of water and other liquids. Each fasting method of fasting serves a purpose and it is up to the individual to gauge what is right for them.

. . .

IN CASE OF PROTEIN FASTING, people withhold the consumption of protein. They fill up on other forms of nutrients such as carbs and fat (in controlled measures).

IN PROTEIN FASTING, people reduce the consumption of protein to 20 grams in one day of the week. The idea behind protein fast is to encourage the occurrence of autophagy in the body. Additionally, this type of fasting helps you burn fat without turning to OMAD or other forms of fasting.

IT SHOULD BE UNDERSTOOD that if you are adopting protein fasting, then process of autophagy takes a longer time to show its results as compared to OMAD.

WITH OMAD, you are going to see the results quickly, as you are expunging all unnecessary compounds from your diet for most of the day. Even when you eat, you are eating a controlled diet that consists of high fats and low carbs.

ALTERNATE-DAY FASTING

ALTERNATE-DAY FASTING or ADF (we do love our acronyms) is another form of intermittent fasting.

THE FOUNDATION of this fasting is based on the idea that you fast on one day, then you eat what you feel like on the next day. Basically, it is a way to halve what you eat on a daily basis.

. . .

On the days that you are fasting, you are allowed to have calorie-free beverages. Because Alternate-Day Fasting does not entirely cut your supply of food, many people find it easier to work with than other forms of fasting.

Water Fasting

Water fasting is a fairly common practice of fasting. In fact, it has been present throughout history in some form or another.

When you are ready to do an extended water fast, one of the things you should remember is to practice with other fasting types before you try on the water fast.

Which is why I recommend that you begin with an OMAD fast. Keep the fast going on for about 2 – 3 weeks before you begin to try out an extended water fast.

Another thing to remember is that you need to take it easy on yourself before you begin the fast. This means that you should not subject yourself to stressful situations. One of the ways to do that is by making sure that you are not going to your job when you are fasting. You should ideally focus on taking a couple of days of for yourself (if you can) or perhaps try out your fast during your vacation.

Another factor that you should focus on is your breathing. When you take short breaths, then your body engages in a flight or fight response. Your brain thinks that you are about to experience something dangerous. This is why most breathing exercises involves slow

AUTOPHAGY

deep breaths. Practice breathing slowly so that you train your body to not enter into a flight or fight condition. This could cause stress to your body, which eventually leads to the consumption of more energy. This means you get hungry really fast.

WHEN YOU ARE READY, you need to go on an extended water fast for at least 2 – 3 days.

DURING THE FAST ITSELF, you are supposed to take in as many essential minerals as possible. For this reason, stick to mineral water. Ensure that you hydrate yourself in the morning so that you can fill up the electrolytes in your system. One of the best ways to go through with this diet is to have positive people around you. They motivate you and make you feel good about your fast. This in turn has positive effects on the body and the mind. You feel less stressed. You feel more motivated. More importantly, you feel happy. After all, you shouldn't be depressed about fasting!

72-HOUR FASTING

I LOVE SCIENCE. Okay, perhaps I should explain that before I go any further.

YOU SEE, I believe in the power of science to back up the tons of research conducted on intermittent fasting and autophagy. I love how we can explain what is happening on a detailed basis if we want to. Moreover, I like how we can break down the science to make it understandable for everyone.

. . .

So, why am I talking about science and putting it under a positive light? No, I did not have a sudden epiphany.

The reason why I brought up science is that most people find it difficult to believe that a 72-hour fasting can be beneficial to them. They are under the impression that no one can do it. However, they forget the resiliency of the human body.

We are able to adapt to anything and one of the ways we can show that is by controlling our mindset about eating. You see, eating is something we do on a daily basis. It is not easy to give up on the habits that we are depending on sustaining us.

According to research conducted at the University of Southern California, abstaining from having food for even two days can result in regenerative properties for the immune system and help the body fight infections better.[1]

The investigation took place on two- and four-day fasting on humans (not mice this time), and the results showed that not only does the immune system get stronger, but the body gets rid of damaged parts better.

That is the benefit of going on a 72-hour fast.

When you are under this fast, you have to make sure that you understand what you can consume and what you cannot. For example, coffee and liquids such as Apple Cider Vinegar is known to curb hunger. However, you cannot just take any coffee. You are only

AUTOPHAGY

allowed to consume plain coffee. No cream or sugar. So say goodbye to the double espresso chocolate cream caramel Frappuccino.

ONE OF THE questions people ask about this fasting is why it is necessary when we already have a 12-hour is fasting. For one, your body is digesting food 12 hours after you have consumed it. So, biologically speaking, you haven't yet entered into a state of fasting yet.

THAT IS WHY, when you are on a 72-hour fast, you make sure that you let your body complete its digestion process and get rid of the last remains of the food in your body.

ONCE YOUR BODY has completed digesting everything, you let it fast for a prolonged period of time.

HOWEVER, remember that you cannot simply enter into a 72-hour fasting.

YOU HAVE to begin with OMAD fasting and keep at it for at least 2 to 3 weeks. Once your body gets used to OMAD fasting, then you are ready to take it to the next step.

I WOULD ALSO RECOMMEND that you get comfortable with water fasting for 24 hours. This will help your body prepare itself for longer fasting periods. You will have a better time getting comfortable with the 72-hour fast and you are less likely to suffer hunger pangs.

. . .

OF COURSE, the big question is what you can and cannot drink while fasting. Apart from water fasting (where you have to focus on taking in mainly mineral water), here are some of the liquid that you can consume (no matter what fasting you have decided to adopt).

LIQUIDS ***to Consume While Fasting***
    Water

I THINK many readers might respond by saying "duh!" upon reading that water is part of the list of liquids that you can drink while fasting.

I AGREE. Hydrating yourself is essential during the fasting process. Nevertheless, you need to be aware of what water you are about to consume during the fast.

IDEALLY, you should be taking mineral water. This is because there is a reason they are called mineral water. They contain essential compounds such as sodium that are vital for your body.

TEA

TEA IS AN INCREDIBLY vital part of any fast. You have various tea options to choose from but I would recommend sticking to ==black tea, green tea, chamomile tea or oolong tea.==

ONE OF THE main reasons for having tea is that it can reduce the levels of hunger in the body in addition to providing essential antioxidants.

. . .

WHEN YOU ARE HAVING any of the tea mentioned above, do make sure that you are not adding anything to it. You should stick to plain tea. No cream or sugar or even honey. If you need a dose of caffeine, then note that tea has a higher level of caffeine than coffee.

COFFEE

WITHOUT ANY ADDITIVES, coffee is a great drink to include in your diet. It provides your body with antioxidants. This in-turn helps your body repair damage caused to your cells by free radicals, which can cause some rather unpleasant side effects as well as we had seen earlier. There have also been studies that show that coffee contributes to an increase in the production of ketones.

ONE OF THE main benefits of coffee is that is a calorie-free beverage. That is why, it not only helps you remain active when you require it, but it does not add any additional calories that you should be worried about.

A FAIR WARNING HOWEVER. Coffee might have some adverse effects. People who are not used to caffeine (or even in those who are regular caffeine-drinkers), coffee is known to produce reactions such as an upset stomach, acid reflux, or even carpal tunnel syndrome. (That name sounds dangerous, but it is simply a numbing feeling at the tips of your fingers that is not fatal yet uncomfortable nonetheless.)

TRY NOT to consume Bulletproof coffee during your fast. This is a coffee that is made using a combination of coffee, coconut oil, and unsalted butter. Because of the ingredients involved in making it, the drink might contain a fairly high level of calories. This means that having the coffee might result in the break of your fast.

One final note: no sugar or cream in your coffee. You have to drink it plain.

Baking Soda

Because you are fasting and you are mainly using liquids to sustain you for the duration of the fast, you tend to urinate quite frequently. This means that you have to make sure that you are maintaining the levels of electrolytes in your body.

One of the main reasons for using baking soda is that it consists of sodium bicarbonate. This is important for getting sodium into your body. This helps you build up the electrolytes in your body. Ideally, you should be adding about one teaspoon of sodium bicarbonate in a glass of water. A fair warning though: baking soda does not really taste that great. Its taste is one of the reasons why people do not usually add it as part of their fast.

Glauber's Salts

If your main aim of fasting is to promote your health and assist your body with cleaning the cells, then you need to have Glauber's salts.

Commonly referred to as sodium sulfate decahydrate by the scientific community, Glauber's salt is a type of mild laxative. It helps in cleaning out the digestive tract and getting rid of constipation. You only need to add about 10 grams of Grauber's salt in a glass of water.

Apple Cider Vinegar

The use of apple cider vinegar is not a recent discovery. For many years, people have been using ACV to treat a wide variety of ailments.

Just like coffee, ACV does not have any calories in it. But the benefits it provides can help you with your fasting in many ways. For one, it helps you maintain your electrolytes. Secondly, it helps prevent any deficiencies that might arise during your fast. This is because ACV contains essential elements in it such as iron, magnesium, and potassium. ACV is also known to clean your gut by killing any harmful bacteria that might be present there.

Finally – and probably one of the most important reasons – ACV staves off hunger really well. It also has a great taste, especially when you add it to sparkling water.

You should make sure that you are not consuming more than 2 tablespoons of ACV at a given time.

Natural Sweeteners

People might often say that having natural sweetener does not cause a lot of problems. However, there are a few things that you should note about natural sweeteners. If you really would like to have them, then you are better off using sweeteners like Stevia over any other type.

If you are getting the sweeteners in powdered form, then make sure you check the label before you use them. The reason is that they may contain maltodextrin (another name for sugar that manufacturers try to use). If you find the ingredients and you still use the sweetener, then it is as good as using sugar.

Another thing to note is that if you are using sweeteners, then take careful note about how your body feels. If you start feeling hungry really soon or if your hunger levels spike, then you are better off avoiding sweeteners altogether. Your hunger levels can spike because your body can detect a false rise in insulin because of the sweetener.

With that, you have so many options to work with when you are fasting. Make sure that you are keeping yourself rehydrated. People often forget that giving the body proper fluids is one of the key factors in making your fast a successful one.

Since we are on the subject of liquids, you might have thought about adding supplements to your drink or water. After all, we did mention natural sweeteners as a replacement for sugar. So, is there something else you can add in water to give you a boost of nutrients?

There are, and we are going to look at a few of them.

Supplement and Demand

. . .

Spirulina

Who knew algae could be a supplement?

That's what spirulina is. It is a type of blue-green algae that is available as a diet supplement. A lot of people like to think of spirulina as a superfood. However, one can either agree or disagree to that depending on their perspective. Needless to say, the supplement does provide some health benefits such as the below.

One of the things that spirulina provides in abundance is vitamins and proteins. This is why, it is ideal for people who are on diet. I would recommend having the supplement along with the liquids that you have planned to consume during the diet.

Activated Charcoal

Yes, you heard that right.

Charcoal provides health benefits as well.

But before you go to the nearest construction site and start munching on some charcoal, let's start with the basics.
  Activated charcoal is different from the regular forms of charcoal that you know of. It comes in a powder form and is specially manufactured for the main purpose of consumption.

. . .

So, what exactly is activated charcoal useful for?

One of the features of activated charcoal is that it has the property to absorb toxin. It has also been used for numerous medical purposes.

Activated charcoal works to treat diarrhea and can also treat the problem of intestinal gas. When you combine it with your fasting, it ensures that your food is digested properly and you do not face problems with your digestion.

Turmeric

Turmeric is a spice that is commonly used in India. In fact, is has been used in their cooking for centuries. If you ask many people in India, they respond by saying that the main reason that they use turmeric is because it is good for the health. They do not know the specifics, but they believe that the spice helps their body in many ways.

Oh, how right they are.

In fact, science has caught up to the claims of our eastern friends.

The reason why turmeric is really healthy is because of the presence of curcumin. Guess what one of the uses of curcumin is? It has strong anti-inflammatory properties.

. . .

THAT IS WHY, in order to prevent inflammation and make sure that your fasting is engaged in the process of activating autophagy, turmeric is a great addition to your diet. Have a turmeric drink is an excellent way to add the right substances into your body during your fast.

TURMERIC IS ALSO KNOWN to improve the antioxidant properties of the body. This way, you lower the chances of getting oxidative stress considerably. Aside from that, it is believed to assist with improvements in brain functions and lower the risk of brain diseases.

IN ALL, turmeric makes sure you avoid inflammation and oxidative stress in the body while also improving brain functions. Due to this, you feel more focused, less stressed, and more active during your fasting.

ONE OF THE ways that you can take turmeric is through the many supplements available in the market. Do make sure you conduct research on turmeric supplement you are taking and ensure that you have read the reviews about the product before you make your purchase, though. It helps you to make an informed purchase decision.

BRING *in the Acid*

THERE ARE many supplements to choose from in the market.

. . .

You need to get yourself one that your body can digest easily. It should also be able to be absorbed by the body, else there is no point in taking the supplement at all in the first place.

However, how can you ensure that the supplement you are taking is absorbed by the body? You use vinegar and water.

What you have to do is mix equal parts vinegar and water in a glass. You then take your pills and drop them into the liquid mixture. You then wait for no more than 40 minutes.

If the pills dissolve within those 40 minutes, then you can continue taking the pills. However, if you notice that the pills haven't dissolved even after 40 minutes, then you have to get rid of them.

They are not going to be digested by your body.

Once you have confirmed whether the pill can dissolve in the mixture, you can safely consume it.

Sleep Time

Simply eating the right diet, liquids, and supplements are not enough for your fasting. You need more.

You need to give your body a little rest. But apart from rest, there are numerous benefits that sleep can provide to your body.

- When you sleep, your body repairs any damaged cells, works on developing your immune system, and performs various functions that it could not when your body was active.
- Furthermore, sleep helps to reduce stress. This is important because the more stress you have, the more it affects your fasting. You end up getting hungry really fast and then it becomes difficult for you to maintain your fast. Reducing the levels of stress is particularly important during the 72-hour fasting routine. This is because you are going to go for a long time without food and you need your brain to remain calm and distressed.
- Autophagy helps in inflammation. So does sleep. When you are fasting and you activate autophagy, you need to get a good night's sleep to make sure that you are allowing autophagy to work properly in your body.
- If you are fasting to lose weight, then you need to make sure that you get a good night's sleep. This is because lack of sleep affects the hormones in the body. When your hormones are affected, it becomes difficult for your body to focus on your weight.
- Want to maintain your appetite? Get some sleep. Without proper sleep, the hormones ghrelin and leptin (responsible for appetite) are disrupted. This means that you end up feeling much hungrier than you should.
- Make sure that you head to bed the same time every night. Your body loves routines when it comes to sleep. This is because it is planning ahead. It knows that you are going to sleep at a particular time and so it adjusts its functions accordingly. This allows your body to prepare for the night. If you keep changing your sleep schedules, you are going to cause more harm than good. How much harm? Well, let's just look a few shall we?
- Changing sleep schedules leads to increase in diabetes and heart diseases.

- More importantly, your body's insulin levels are disrupted, making it difficult for you to fast properly. Changing sleep schedules has also been known to create a resistance to insulin. This means that insulin does not properly convert the sugar into energy in your body.
- Frequently changing your sleep patterns increases your Body Mass Index, or BMI. In other words, you begin to gain more weight.

Having proper sleep is essential during your fasting. It goes hand-in-hand with our diet, your exercises, and everything you do during the period of food-deprivation.

Having concluded that sleep is important, the next set of questions that come to you are:

- What about during your waking hours?
- Is there something you can do to improve your body while you are awake?
- Is exercising possible? Is there anything else that you should be doing besides exercising?

You can do two things: 1) exercise, which we have already mentioned before, and 2) go to the sauna. You read that right.

Gonna Go To the Sauna

. . .

AUTOPHAGY

Recently, a surprising discovery was made in the world of intermittent fasting.

When you are using any of the ways for your intermittent fasting process, you can always choose to combine it with a session at the sauna.

They make a powerful combination.

How?

When you are in a sauna, your body experiences a process that the medical community calls "hyperthermic conditioning." During this process, the infrared heat in the sauna causes certain changes in the body. These changes help the body to burn more calories and improve the metabolic processes. As you can see, these are some of the things that we are trying to achieve through intermittent fasting.

When you combine your time at the sauna and the benefits gained from intermittent fasting, you ensure that the two processes work together to provide even greater benefits to your body. In fact, here are some of the other benefits gained from heading over to the sauna while fasting:

- When you are losing fat, you also need to lose the water weight present in your body. You are practically sweating inside a sauna. This removes the water weight, preparing your body for weight loss.
- It has been recorded that you can burn as much as 300 calories in a short sauna session. As you are already

restricting your diet during fasting, heading over to the sauna only serves to boost your weight loss targets.
- Because you sweat profusely in a sauna, you flush out toxins from your system. This, when combined with autophagy, becomes a powerful way to cleanse your body.

Getting Worked Up

Working out and exercising benefit your fasting in many ways.

When you are fasting, your body is ready to burn the fat in your body. But when add in exercises and workout routines during your fasting period, then it increases the rate at which your body burns fat tremendously. According to research, if you workout during fasting, then your body burns up to 20 percent more fat than usual.

Plus, you also lower your insulin levels faster when you exercise. This is because you are using up energy at an increases state. Your body actually demands more energy and eventually turns out that you are adding to your body through your keto diet for that purpose.

And let us not forget the fact that exercising helps you improve your muscles. Combine it with the fat-reducing properties of a keto diet, then you can develop your body faster.

But what are the exercises that you can do while you are fasting.

. . .

DO NOTE a few important points before you begin working out:

- Do not exercise for more than 60 minutes in a day. This is to ensure that you do not push your body too much. You are fasting and you need to prevent yourself from getting too hungry.
- If you feel dizzy or weak at any point during your exercises, then do not think of having water and returning to your exercises. Stop immediately and come back to it the next day. Give your body time to adjust to exercising while it is undergoing a fasting session. Do not push it in order to get results.
- You might not notice changes immediately. This is probably true for all workouts. However, when you are fasting, the results take a bit longer to show. Ideally, you might start noticing physical changes after 2 weeks of fasting. This is completely normal and it has got nothing to do with your body.
- Always remember to start small. Try and check the extent to which you can exercise. Start with small number of repetitions and gradually increase as you get accustomed to the exercise. Do not use regular exercise tips because they are not meant for fasting.
- Hydrate yourself properly. Make sure you are sticking to your keto diet so that you supply your body with high fats that it can use during exercises. You can choose to have coffee an hour or so before you work out should you feel like it, but make sure it is plain coffee.
- Make sure you choose the workout based on the type of food you are consuming. If you do not have carbs in your diet, then you should try and avoid high-intensity workout.

THE FIRST STEP that you should take is that you need to start off easy. You need to use simple exercises such as brisk walking or cycling slowly. These exercises prepare the body for the more intense workouts.

THEN, move on to medium intensity exercises. This way, you can keep your body fit and make sure that you can continue with your fasting without any problems.

WHILE YOU ARE WORKING OUT, make sure that you are paying attention to your body so that you can notice signs or dehydration or of low-blood sugar (which usually is the case when you begin to feel dizzy).

Not as Intense

ONE OF THE types of exercises that you can do is a low intensity cardio.

WHAT IS the benefit of this cardio?

WELL FOR ONE, low intensity cardio does not lead to any injury, extreme exhaustion, or even a burnout. This means that you can work up a good sweat, but your will still have time to perform other tasks (in this case, fasting).

IS THERE a way to know whether you are performing your exercise at low intensity cardio? Sure, there is.

. . .

WHEN YOU ARE EXERCISING at a low intensity, then you are performing at a level that uses 60% to 80% of your maximum heart rate. When you reach that level, you can perform your workouts for longer periods and at the same time, build your endurance as well.

HOW EXACTLY CAN you measure your maximum heart rate? Simple. You simply take your age and subtract it from the number 220. To calculate the heart rate ideal for your workout, take 60% of the resulting number and then calculate 80% of the number. You should aim for the heart rate between the two numbers.

LET me explain this with an example.

SAY that you are 30 years old. Your maximum heart rate is 190. Now, you are going to calculate the heart rate ideal for your workout. Let's first calculate 60% of 190 and then 80% of 190.

YOU GET TWO NUMBERS: 114 and 152. This means that when you are working out, you should ideally keep your heart rate between 114 and 152.

WHEN YOU GET A NUMBER, then you will be able to easily check your heart rate during your workout and then see if you are within the range that you calculated for yourself.

ONCE YOU HAVE FIGURED out how to continue with your exercises, it becomes easier for you to keep going for at least 20 to 30 minutes, if not an entire hour.

. . .

THOMAS HAWTHORN

Exercise and Autophagy

mTor.

That word might not really mean much to you. But you still need to know why it is important in the context of autophagy.

Let us say that mTor is bad news. In fact, the word sounds like the name of a Terminator. And it might as well be because mTor is related to the "terminator" of diseases; cancer.

mTor is a type of protein that is most commonly found in certain types of cancer. This means that you have to ideally aim to block of the protein before it causes further harm.

When you exercise, you end up blocking the mTor pathways. This in turn generates a mild form of autophagy. However, here is where it makes a whole lot of difference.

You are already fasting. This means that you have already reached a point where you have activated autophagy. So even the little autophagy that exercising activates is more like a boost to the process already occurring in your body.

The benefit does not go in one direction. This means that it is not just exercising that benefits autophagy, but autophagy benefitting your workouts as well.

. . .

AUTOPHAGY DOES NOT CONTRIBUTE to direct muscles development. But it builds up the resistance in the tissues. This means that your body can resist against catabolic stressors during your exercises. What exactly are catabolic stressors?

IT IS A TYPE OF STRESS. This means that it is bad news.

WHAT HAPPENS IS that when you are exercising, your body is obviously experiencing the result of your workouts. One of the results is the effect exercise has on your metabolism.

WHEN YOU ARE WORKING OUT, you disrupt the metabolic state in your body. This disruption of the metabolism of the body is termed as catabolic stressors. This means that apart from exercising, you might need a bit more help from another source.

ONE OF THE ways to bring back the metabolism back to normality is through autophagy.

THROUGH THIS COMPLEMENTARY relationship between exercise and autophagy, you can continue working out without any adverse changes to your body.

AGE WELL

REMEMBER when we say how autophagy can provide your body with anti-aging benefits? Exercise does the same as well.

. . .

IN FACT, according to a study published in the University of Birmingham, exercise is known to keep the body young and healthy. So, this is how it happens.

WHEN YOU EXERCISE, you pump blood to different parts of the body. This allows the tissues and cells to remain active and receive all the nutrients in the blood. When the cells receive all of the nutrients that you supply to them, then they do not age or die off very easily. Those that die off are automatically removed by the process of autophagy. In this way, you have younger cells and, at the same time, you are getting rid of older cells.

APART FROM WORKING on the cells, exercise also works on your muscles. Whether you are a man or a woman, exercise provides the same set of benefits to you. You gain a more active lifestyle and this contributes to a younger body that carries well into your 40s, 50s and beyond.

EXERCISE IS a potent way to recharge your body and unlock its full potential.

REMEMBER when we talked about getting a good night's sleep? One of the ways that you can improve the quality of your sleep and ensure that you head to bed at the same time every night is by exercising regularly.

THIS IS BECAUSE, when you engage in physical activities, you end up making a big contribution towards a restful and sound sleep. Moreover, apart from increasing the quality of the sleep you receive, exercise also increases the quantity of sleep. When you are physically active, you have to spend the energy in your body. When you expend that energy, you feel tired and that helps your body prepare itself for a state of rest. This is why, when you have a day filled with physical activities, you feel like crashing on the bed.

THAT IS nothing but your body waiting for you to head to bed so that it can begin to use its energy reserves and keep you fresh for when you wake up.

Meet the Resistance!

WE HAD ALREADY TALKED about cardio exercises and how they can benefit your body in many ways. There is another form of exercise that you could adopt into your fasting routine: resistance exercise.

WHAT DOES this exercise entail and just what sort of benefits are you looking at by performing these exercises?

RESISTANCE EXERCISES, or resistance training, refers to those exercises that allow the muscles to apply force against a source of resistance. Because of this force, the muscles tend to increase in strength, mass, tone, and endurance. With such an expectation in mind, the external force that your body receives can be added through various means such as weights, bars, dumbbells or even your own body weight.

THERE ARE several types of resistance exercises. You might have heard of weight lifting, which is one of the popular methods of resistance exercise. However, that is an example of a high-intensity work out and something you should not be including in your routine if you are fasting.

You could try some low-intensity resistance exercise that could help you with your work out requirements.

Some of the low-intensity exercises that you can do are:

- Push-ups
- Dumbbells (make sure that you are not trying to lift extremely heavy weights. You do not want to tire yourself out too much at this point)
- Squats
- Crunches

Simply allowing yourself to perform some of these exercises will lead to a whole lot of benefits to your body.

So, what are the benefits you receive from resistance training? Quite a lot, to be honest.

- For one, you get to improve your muscle tone and strength. This leads to the overall development of your muscles.
- As you grow older, you might find out that your flexibility and balance could fail you. This is because your muscles are not trained to stretch or bear the brunt of an expanding force. Resistance exercises allow you to be flexible and agile, giving you greater balance and increased vitality.
- Cognition tends to drop as you grow older. When you take part in resistance exercises, then you improve your brain's

ability to retain information and develop its cognitive abilities.
- Resistance training also improves your moods, lowers your stress levels, and prevents you from entering into a state of depression.
- Your posture is always at risk as you grow older. Your spine tends to bend forward, either because of the way you sit at work or because you are used to stooping while walking. Regardless of the situation, you may find yourself having a poor angle for your body when it is upright. When you practice resistance exercises, then you improve your posture drastically. You end up walking straighter. This has an effect on your level of confidence. Research has shown that by simply walking straight, you psychologically convince yourself that you are more confident.

AUTOPHAGY SUCCESS STORIES

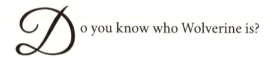o you know who Wolverine is?

YES, that guy who had adamantium claws come out of his hands and bad attitude, was a part of the X-Men, and took out enemy mutants.

OH, wait, you know what? I think you might know the person behind the character. So, let me try asking the question again and perhaps you might have a positive response.

Do you know who Hugh Jackman is?

THAT'S RIGHT. Now, that name might sound a bit more familiar.

. . .

AUTOPHAGY

IF YOU GOOGLE the terms "Hugh Jackman" and "Wolverine," chances are that you may spot a picture of the actor showing off his ripped body for the role. Furthermore, there is also a possibility that you may find the term "intermittent fasting."

Why is that?

TURNS OUT, the actor combined workout sessions with intermittent fasting to reach the body type that he was aiming for. And it shows.

HUGH JACKMAN IS JUST one of many people who have found success using the intermittent fasting diet.

PEOPLE often incorporate intermittent fasting or keto diet into their lives in a way that suits them best. They then form new habits to achieve the health goals that they have set up for themselves. In the case of Hugh Jackman, it was getting his body so ripped that it actually looks like it can deflect real arrows.

IN THE CASE of Gina Lassales, meanwhile, it was losing weight.

IF YOUR NEXT thought goes along the lines of "Who is this person?", then I can definitely understand the confusion.

YOU SEE, at one point in time, Gina used to weigh around 300 pounds.

SHE WANTED to do something about it and found out that traditional methods of diets were not working for her. She decided that she would overhaul her diet. Eventually, Gina discovered a Facebook group that was focused on keto diet. She ended up losing nearly 180 pounds of weight and turned her life around. She became happier and more active. She changed her life. And the rest, as hey say, is history.

THE ABOVE EXAMPLES are just two of the many people who have made major improvements in their lives by adopting a keto diet or going through intermittent fasting. Now, let us try and look at another example.

Do you know what Keto Karma is?

TO BE FAIR, I might have asked the question wrong just to see if the name rings and bells.

THE RIGHT QUESTION SHOULD BE: Do you know *who* Keto Karma is?

FOR MANY YEARS, Suzanne Ryan was struggling with obesity. This led her to develop mental health problems, such as depression, anxiety, and hopelessness that not just worsened her situation but also affected the way she saw herself. At the time, Suzanne was struggling with emotional problems, and food became her source of comfort. Eventually, she became addicted to food as a source of comfort. This did not help her situation because she entered a cycle where she would eat to gain comfort, gain weight, become emotional about her weight gain, and then go back to eating more.

IN THE YEARS THAT FOLLOWED, Suzanne tried all kinds of weight loss programs. She tried becoming a vegetarian and sticking to a non-meat diet. However, that had little effect on her body. She tried juicing, but it did not provide her the results that she was looking for. And despite the other methods that she also tried, the difference was either minimal or not showing at all.

WHEN DIETS DID NOT WORK, Suzanne turned to supplements. She experimented with a few, but once again, the changes were either too dismal to notice or not existing at all.

THAT WAS when Suzanne found keto diet. By that time, she was over 300 pounds, married, and had just given birth to her daughter. She realized that taking care of her child was exerting a toll on her, and she was unable to remain active for long.

OF COURSE, her initial venture into keto diet was difficult. Her dependency on carbs were really high, and this developed a high-carb "craze" in her life. She almost gave up on the diet, but she stuck to it because she did notice changes in her life.

EVENTUALLY, Suzanne lost a total of 120 pounds through the program. Since then, she hasn't changed her mind about the diet. She turned her lessons with keto diet into her own book and became known to her readers as Keto Karma.

AUTOPHAGY Is MORE than Just a Fad

IT IS A SCIENTIFICALLY PROVEN process that your body actually makes use of. However, with the lifestyle that we lead, we do not have enough opportunities to activate the process. We have to face the stress of daily life. Our food habits are not exactly what one would call healthy and even if we are sticking to vegetables and fruits, we are unsure which of those vegetables and fruits have high carbs. Oh yes, the stuff you consider healthy might actually have carbs in them.

THAT IS where autophagy comes into play.

THE LIFESTYLE that revolves around intermittent fasting, keto diet, and autophagy is one that has a specific set of goals. Each of them is backed up by science so that you receive the greatest benefits in your life as you adopt newer and healthier habits into your life.

OF COURSE, the road to gaining a good life is packed with challenges. But what isn't?

IF YOU HAVE DECIDED to head to the gym to build your muscles, then you are going to experience muscle pains, cramps, and stiffness for the first week or so. You might find it difficult to even lift your hands up to perform a simple action. Still, you must persist. You know that at the end of your journey, you are going to be rewarded with a body that is healthy, fit, and probably packed with muscles as well!

AFTERWORD

Forget about juice cleanses and other forms of diet that you have heard of.

Autophagy is the next step towards a healthier life.

And that is not just me saying it. According to the National Institute of Diabetes and Digestive and Kidney Diseases, autophagy has already been known to protect individuals against cancer and other diseases. Further research has shown that the process also plays a vital role in the management of conditions such as obesity and type 2 diabetes.

The question you have to ask here should not be focused on why medicine and science is trying to show the benefits of autophagy. The question should be, "What took them so long?" But progress takes place through small steps.

We learn. We discover. We evolve.

This is the same with science as well.

AFTERWORD

It learns. It adapts. It changes perspectives.

With autophagy, perspectives are slowly changing about the process. At one point, people used to believe that they were just about to see another diet fad being promoted by individuals who probably did not have any clue about the biological impacts of such fads.

Today, people are more informed. They want to know more about what they are doing. They want to understand - partially, if not fully - the mechanics behind what a particular diet, fast, or technique does.

Thankfully, autophagy has the answers for you. Leaning on heavy research into the body and the science behind proper dieting, fasting, and fitness, autophagy combines what we know and creates a body of work designed to help people turn their life around.

Does autophagy improve the health?

That question was posed to scientists. In a report done by the BBC, the news network wanted to find out what scientists actually think about autophagy. Is this just another hoax? Is it a research that is only made to fit a large group of companies? Does it involve taking a specific set of drugs so that it can boost the sales of certain pharmaceuticals?

Dr. David Rubinsztein, a professor of molecular neurogenetics at the UK Dementia Research Institute, has been examining the research conducted on mice.[1] According to him, the evidence from the research seems to show that autophagy indeed does improve the health of the rodents.

He is not the only one from the scientific and medical community making his voice vocal. Let us not forget the research conducted by Dr. Yoshinori Ohsumi that earned a Nobel Prize. People are always

AFTERWORD

looking for ways to bring better changes to their lives. In today's world of fast-food trends, that just seems to keep on creating new products (in fact, the world thinks that bigger is better). You have pizzas made with 2 pounds of dough and got enough cheese to feed an army of mice! You have burgers that look like they can feed at least 20 people for an entire day as well!

All of these trends keep on building up. The food industry is all about competition. It focuses on who makes the biggest, most innovative, most complex food out there. Every business aims to stand out. But in doing so, they create unhealthy habits for the people.

And it is not just the habits that are getting affected. People spend so much to enjoy a bit of the "new and unique stuff." So, in the end, you have people losing the quality of their health, as well as their money simply to enjoy something that is considerably unhealthier than anything that they have ever tried before.

It is because of the abundance of so many unhealthy food trends that people have discovered that there is a lack of trends that promote good food. Even among the food trends, after all, not many are reliable.

This is where autophagy comes in. The scientific community has realized the effects that unhealthy eating has on people. Their aim to bring autophagy into the lives of everyone is a way for them to introduce new habits.

When all is said and done, autophagy is a truly reliable process in the body, and activating it brings in a host of benefits.

So, I think it is time for us to begin making changes into our lives.

It is time to take our health into our own hands.

AFTERWORD

It is time to bring a wonderful change into our lives.

And, if at any point, you do not understand what you are doing, worry not. That is what this book is made for.

It is called *Autophagy for Beginners*, after all.

With that, I wish you all a good life.

NOTES

2. AUTOPHAGY IN PLAIN ENGLISH

1. The Nobel Prize. (2016). The Nobel Prize in Physiology or Medicine 2016. Retrieved from https://www.nobelprize.org/prizes/medicine/2016/press-release/

5. OXIDATIVE STRESS AND YOUR HORMONES

1. Szalay, J. (2016). What Are Free Radicals?. Retrieved from https://www.livescience.com/54901-free-radicals.html

10. AUTOPHAGY LIFESTYLE: HOW TO INCORPORATE FASTING INTO YOUR DAILY LIFE

1. Garsema, E. (2017). Scientifically designed fasting diet lowers risks for major diseases. Retrieved from https://news.usc.edu/116479/scientifically-designed-fasting-diet-lowers-risks-for-major-diseases/

AFTERWORD

1. University of Cambridge. (2019). Blood pressure drug shows promise for treating Parkinson's and dementia in animal studies. Retrieved from https://www.cam.ac.uk/research/news/blood-pressure-drug-shows-promise-for-treating-parkinsons-and-dementia-in-animal-studies

Made in United States
Orlando, FL
21 April 2022